Practical Dispensing

A hand-book intended for those engaged in ophthalmic dispensing and allied activities.

Antony I Griffiths, FBDO(Hons), Dip.Dist.Ed.

published by:

The Association of British Dispensing Opticians
6 Hurlingham Business Park
Sulivan Road
London
SW6 3DU

printed by:

UNWIN BROTHERS LIMITED
The Gresham Press, Old Woking, Surrey
A Member of the Martins Printing Group

ISBN 0-900099-33-x

First Edition	**1995**
Second Edition	**1997**
Third Edition	**2000**

Contents

PREFACE

When you start to write a book all sorts of questions arise. What should be included? What should be omitted? To what depth do we need to go? Who is going to read the book?

As the chapters start to take shape - some easily, some with great difficulty - other questions come into mind. Why am I doing this? Will I ever be able to finish?

As the whole thing progresses despite the anxieties it becomes patently obvious that many of the things written are already becoming out of date, especially those things relating to the availability of lenses. No sooner have you decided that a particular lens design or material is the greatest thing since sliced bread than somebody brings out a better one, or at least a newer one.

I originally felt that I should be eternally grateful if anyone at all reads this book, as indeed I am. I was therefore somewhat surprised, but nevertheless delighted that the first edition was well received, both at home and overseas.

In the light of this encouragement I have tried to eliminate previous errors and omissions, as well as endeavouring to make some areas clearer.

I can only hope that I have succeeded.

Tony Griffiths

March 2000

1. INTRODUCTION

Most books on optics commence with an historical background to the topic under consideration. Where does history begin? When you reach a certain tender age, history has a nasty habit of catching up with you. History is also very slanted. It is usually only seen and reported from one viewpoint. On this premise I will therefore give some background history to Practical Dispensing.

In the past, and still today to some extent a job was learned by the technique known as "sitting with Nelly". This meant that the "apprentice" sat alongside someone who had been doing the job for many many years and who had no doubt seen many apprentices come and go. Nelly would carry out the routines required to perform her [Nelly could of course be male] functions and the apprentice would observe and gradually copy these routines. Sometimes words of explanation would emanate from Nellie's lips, but as often as not Nelly would not know why she performed in the way that she did, or else she wasn't telling.

As time passed the apprentice became more efficient and self-sufficient, eventually either becoming a clone of Nelly or more usually progressing up the ladder via other Nellys.

Dispensing Optics used to follow similar principles with a trainee sitting in with an assistant manager and possibly a manager of a dispensing practice until after many years of patient, or impatient, observation he would be allowed to take over some of the functions of an assistant and eventually become a fully fledged assistant with aspirations of becoming a manager.

Today in most optical establishments trainee dispensing opticians receive more formal training, with the larger organisations boasting training departments and training officers. For those trainees who opt for the distance learning approach to qualification there is the combination of theoretical work via the correspondence courses of the Association of British Dispensing Opticians, plus the practical daily involvement in the branch. In addition of course students also attend college for a brief spell of face to face tuition.

My early days were spent in the "sitting with Nelly" routine and as a result much of my initial dispensing practice involved a rule-of-thumb technique adopted and adapted from my ophthalmic manager. However after a relatively short period of time I began to question why he did some of the things and because he didn't know the answers, but knew a man who did, he suggested that I approached the then Association of Dispensing Opticians about their correspondence courses for dispensers. The rest is history.

In my early days of study I found that many of the topics I was interested in were spread about in various textbooks and journals which I couldn't afford. Amongst the most often perused where 'Ophthalmic Prescription Work' by Bennett & Blumlein, 'The Principles of Ophthalmic Lenses' by Mo Jalie, 'Optics' by Fincham & Freeman, 'Spectacle Fitting and Optical Dispensing' by Sasieni, and in later years 'Optics' by Tunnacliffe & Hirst, 'System for Ophthalmic Dispensing' by Brooks & Borish and many more. I have tried to collect together my gleanings from these tomes and to assemble them together in one place.

In the chapters that follow I will attempt to combine the rules of thumb learned by watching and observing with the theoretical knowledge gained from the A.D.O. correspondence courses.

It is my hope that you will be able to put the former to good use but will continue with your searching to understand the reasoning behind the practical aspects of dispensing.

Chapter Two deals with my version of history relating to Optics as I know it.

2. HISTORY

Two very important events took place on 5th July 1948. The first being my 11th birthday. The second was the introduction of the National Health Service.

At that time amongst other things opticians were recognised as a profession enabled to provide ophthalmic services to the British public. They were in fact enshrined in the Optician's Act as the Supplementary Ophthalmic Services.

The Government of the day carried out some research and consulted with interested parties as to the possible extent of the services that would need to be provided. As with Governments before it, and no doubt for ever more, it decided that the estimates were excessive and consequently cut everything in two. The Hospital Eye Service was to provide the major part of the service, with opticians destined to play a supporting role. Hence the title Supplementary Ophthalmic Services.

It turned out in fact that demand exceeded everybody's expectations. With free sight-tests and glasses, members of the public were collecting their forms O.S.C.1 [Doctor's recommendation] and popping along to the local optician and ordering a new pair of spectacles. Then the next week they were ordering another pair from a different optician. Why not? - They were FREE. The resulting chaos meant that very soon they were having to wait six months to a year for single vision lenses and up to two years for bifocals. A far cry from the 1 hour service being offered today. The prescription houses were completing their orders in date rotation, with uncompleted jobs stacked to the ceiling.

In 1950 the Government introduced charges for glasses for adults. One pound for single vision lenses and two pounds for bifocals and 8s..3d for a 524 frame. Single vision lenses were available in glass only but could be had in either flat or curved form. Bifocals also came in glass but with the option of 24*mm* round fused, 22*mm*, 38*mm* or 45*mm* round solid segments.

There were approximately twenty-five frames available on the NHS including about six for children. There was a choice of:

Section A. Children's Standard Frames

Frame Number	Description
	Plain Nickel
C.127	Pad bridge, short loop end sides
	Nickel Windsor
C.223	Pad bridge, half-covered, curl sides
C.223 H.J.	Pad bridge, high joint, half-covered curl sides
C.227	Pad bridge, short loop end sides
C.253	Pad bridge with additional bridge bar, half-covered curl sides
C.253 H.J.	Pad bridge with additional bridge bar, high joint, half-covered curl sides
To be supplied without charge to children who have not yet attained 16 years of age, and to older boys and girls who are in full-time attendance at a school as defined in the Education Act, 1944 or the Education (Scotland) Act, 1946.	

Section B. Frames other than Children's Standard Frames

Frame Number	Description
221	**Nickel Windsor** Pad bridge, comfort cable curl sides
321 321 H.J. 721 722	**Plain Gold-filled** Pad bridge, comfort cable curl sides Pad bridge, high joint, comfort cable curl sides Half-eye, flat section eyewire, pad bridge, comfort cable curl sides Half-eye, flat section eyewire, pad bridge, zylo-tipped hockey-end sides
421 421 H.J. 422 422 H.J. 423 423 H.J.	**Gold-filled Windsor** Pad bridge, comfort cable curl sides Pad bridge, high joint, comfort cable curl sides Pad bridge, zylo-tipped, hockey-end sides Pad bridge, high joint, zylo-tipped, hockey-end sides Pad bridge, half-covered curl sides Pad bridge, high joint, half-covered curl sides
514 515 524 525 614 615 C525 814 824	**Plastic (Cellulose acetate)*** Regular bridge, with reinforced hockey-end sides Regular bridge, with gold-filled super-comfort curl sides, and reinforced cellulose acetate butts Pad bridge, with reinforced hockey-end sides Pad bridge, with gold-filled super-comfort curl sides, and reinforced cellulose acetate butts Saddle, flush or inset bridge, with reinforced hockey-end sides Saddle, flush or inset bridge, with gold-filled super-comfort curl sides, and reinforced cellulose acetate butts Strong pad bridge, with nickel super-comfort curl sides, and reinforced cellulose acetate butts Half-eye, regular bridge, with reinforced hockey-end sides Half-eye, regular bridge, with reinforced hockey-end sides

* These frames are available under the Service in light brown mottled, dark brown mottled, flesh, crystal, black, and ice blue.

The metal frames were available in chestnut, wine or black. The choice of frames remained unchanged for many years except that because of lack of demand some of the variations disappeared from the list, although I think in about the late 70's a new frame was introduced - the 924 - a plastic 'fashion' frame that was made in three two-tone colours, wine sherry and smoke or was it lavender, and one solid colour brown mottled.

When charges were first introduced the demand for spectacles plummeted overnight. My, how history has a habit of repeating itself. Shortly afterwards the principle of the 'hybrid' was introduced. The idea was that if the cut lenses could be taken out of an NHS frame and fitted into a 'private' frame without re-edging the lens, then the lenses and consequently the charges to the customer could be treated as if they were supplied through the NHS i.e. at a subsidised price. The reclaimable fee from the NHS for such work was however a different matter. Upswept lens shapes or 'supras' were not permitted. With plastic single vision lenses retailing at about thirty pounds per pair and D seg bifocals at fifty pounds per pair in those days it wasn't surprising that few people ventured outside the NHS/hybrid range.

As even the spectacle wearing world became gradually fashion conscious in the 60's new designs of frames became available but they all had this restriction to the basic shape of being panto-round-oval [PRO]. This restraint on design almost resulted in the total downfall of the British frame industry. Continental designers didn't have the same problems and as travel made the world a smaller place so foreign designer frames came into the country and the public clamoured for more.

However before this came about 'fashion' frames were available in cellulose acetate, nitrate and acrylic as well as the odd shell and/or gold frame for the discerning. The choice of colours was by today's standards limited, but the availability of sizes seemed almost limitless. With eye-sizes ranging from 38*mm* to 46*mm* or even a large 48*mm* and DBL's from 16*mm* to 26*mm*. In order to accommodate the new designs and larger eye-sizes lens blanks were also stocked in 60⌀ as well as the normal 55⌀.

I believed then that lens sizes couldn't get any larger because of the weight, thickness and decentration problems that accompanied them. For the young optician of today of course those sizes seem ridiculously small. However because the aim was to dispense the spectacles as close to the patient's eyes as the lashes would permit, the field of view with a 42*mm* round eye was better than that obtained with one of today's much larger eye shapes which probably sits twice as far away. I knew the availability of size and colour of every frame in stock as well as the power range and blank size of all lenses used. But then I probably remembered every patient by name as well.

As both lenses and frames got progressively larger, so new materials, again for lenses as well as frames, became available. And so the public became more dissatisfied with what they could have on the NHS. The fashion element of frames was easier for the public to digest and pay for, but opticians and consequently their patients took longer to see the advantages, both optically and financially, of dispensing quality lenses.

The emphasis of fitting glasses changed from the making of virtually a tailor-made frame with off the peg lenses to that of off the peg frames with tailor-made lenses. This was brought about because of the fact that most 'modern' frames no longer came in a wide range of sizes, but often only two eye-sizes and one bridge size. Whereas the range of available lens types was rapidly increasing. Dispensing challenges revolved around trying to make patients look good in addition to seeing well.

3. SPHERICAL LENSES

Definitions

Before we can talk about spectacle lenses, we must first define some of the terms relating to those lenses. A *spherical lens* is one in which each surface forms part of the surface of a sphere. The radius of curvature of one surface may be infinity, thus making that surface flat or plane.

Spherical surfaces can be either convex or concave. A *convex* surface is one, which is relatively raised at the centre as compared with a *plane* surface, whereas a *concave* surface is relatively depressed at the centre.

Introduction

The lens may be defined as a portion of a transparent substance bounded by two polished surfaces, both of which may be curved, or one only may be curved and the other plane. The curved surfaces may be of a number of different forms, spherical, cylindrical, toroidal, or paraboloidal, but the commonest form of lens is that with spherical surfaces, and the work of this chapter will be limited to this form. Such lenses are usually called **spherical lenses**.

The sign convention

When measuring distances and angles it is useful to give them plus and minus signs to indicate the directions in which the measurements are made. For example, the adoption of such a system or sign convention allows one to state whether an image is upright or inverted just by inspecting the sign attached to its magnitude.

The sign convention used in ophthalmic optics is called *the Cartesian Sign Convention,* which is simply the rectangular co-ordinate system used in co-ordinate or analytical geometry. It derives its name from the French mathematician Rene Descartes (1596-1650) who first devised the system. See the rectangular co-ordinates in Figure 3.1. Measurements along the x-axis are positive to the right of the origin O, and negative to the left. Along the y-axis, measurements upwards are positive and those downwards are negative. This system is adopted by imagining the co-ordinates mounted at each retracting surface so that the x-axis lies along the principal axis, and the origin is at the vertex of the surface, as in Figure 3.2.

Measurements to the right of the vertex **A** are positive and those to the left are negative, whilst measurements upwards above the principal axis are positive and those downwards below the axis are negative.

In addition, signs are applied to the angles between rays and the principal axis, as in Figure 3.3. If, to rotate a ray into the principal axis, it requires an anticlockwise movement of the ray, the angle between the ray and the principal axis is given a positive sign. Rotation of the ray in a clockwise direction into the axis denotes a negative angle.

In applying the sign convention, light is always incident from the left. Should a diagram be drawn with the light incident from the right then the signs for measurements along the principal axis should be reversed. The signs are summarised in Figure 3.3. Rotating the ray into the axis defines the sign of the angle; anti-clockwise rotation is positive. The sign convention is that employed in co-ordinate geometry.

To summarise:

1.   Until a reflecting surface intervenes, light travels from left to right and all refractive indices are positive.

2.   Focal lengths of converging elements are positive; focal lengths of diverging elements are negative.

3.   Ray heights above the axis are positive, below the axis they are negative.

4.   The distance to the right of the vertex of a component [or surface] is positive; to the left it is negative.

5.   The radius of curvature of a surface is positive if its centre lies to the right of the vertex; if to the left of its vertex it is negative.

Fig.3.1 Cartesian rectangular co-ordinates	Fig.3.2 The co-ordinates with the origin at the vertex A of a spherical surface	Fig.3.3 Summary of the sign convention
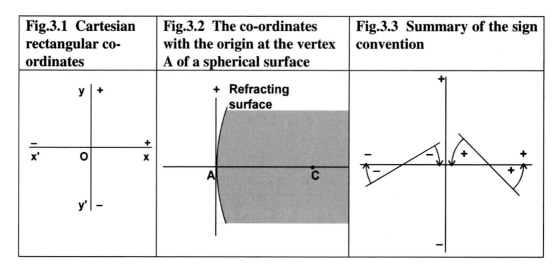		

Forms of Lenses

Thin lenses may be divided into two classes according to the curvature of their surfaces and therefore the effect that they produce on the light. Lenses of the forms shown in Fig.3.4 have either both surfaces or the steeper of the two surfaces convex.

Such lenses, if *thin* and higher refractive index than the surrounding medium, tend to produce convergence of the light - a positive effect. They will therefore be termed **convex, convergent** or **positive**. Lenses having both surfaces or the steeper of the two, surfaces concave, as shown in Fig.3.5, will, under the same conditions, tend to make the light divergent. These will therefore be termed **concave, divergent or negative**.

Fig.3.4 Convex, convergent or positive thin lenses

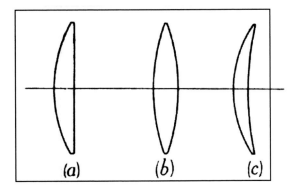

Fig.3.5 Concave, divergent or negative thin lenses

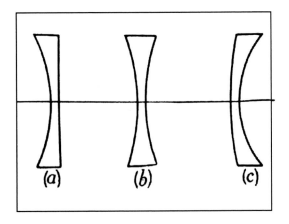

The following terms are applied to the various forms of lenses.

Positive	*Negative*
1. Plano-convex [Fig. 3.4a].	Plano-concave [Fig. 3.5a].
2. Bi-convex [Fig. 3.4b].	Bi-concave [Fig. 3.5b]
3. Equi-convex.	Equi-concave
4. Convex meniscus [Fig. 3.4c].	Concave meniscus [Fig. 3.5c].
5. Convex periscopic.	Concave periscopic.

Periscopic [5] is a term applied to an ophthalmic lens of meniscus form having either one of the surfaces of comparatively small curvature [surface power = 1.25D], the term "meniscus" being used in ophthalmic work for the more "bent" form.

The surface towards the incident light will be called the first surface of the lens, and positions in the space occupied by the incident light will be said to be in front of the lens.

Fig.3.6 represents a section through a biconvex spherical lens, the spheres of which its surfaces are portions having centres at C_1, and C_2, respectively. The straight line C_1C_2 joining the centres of curvature of the two surfaces is called the optical axis of the lens. If one surface is plane, it may be considered as a portion of a sphere of infinite radius, and the optical axis will be the line perpendicular to the plane surface passing through the centre of curvature of the other surface.

Fig.3.6 Optical axis of a lens

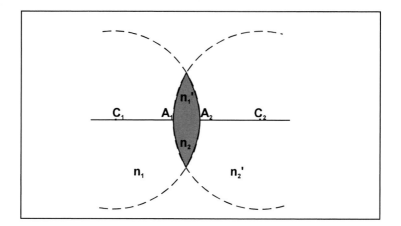

The points A_1 and A_2, where the axis meets the surfaces, are termed the front and back vertex or pole of the lens respectively, and A_1A_2 is the lens thickness. When the lens is so thin that the thickness may be neglected, the common vertex A is the optical centre. Lenses are usually "edged" so that the optical centre coincides with the geometrical centre of the lens aperture. This is not always the case with ophthalmic lenses, such lenses sometimes being "decentred". At the optical centre the two surfaces of the lens are parallel and any rays passing through this point are therefore unchanged in direction. The ray passing through the optical centre is the chief ray from any object point.

Fig.3.7 **Section through a spherical lens. C_1 and C_2 are the centres of curvature. r_1 and r_2 are the radii of curvature. A_1 and A_2 are the front and back vertices.**

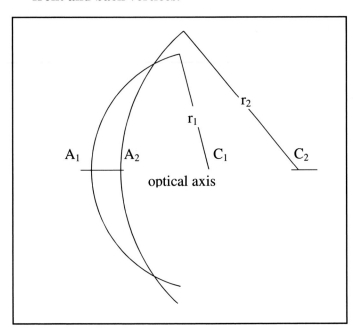

In order for us to quantify the curvature of a surface we need a unit of measurement. The unit chosen is that based on the radius of curvature (*r*), and is in fact the reciprocal of the radius of curvature in metres. Curvature is expressed in units of reciprocal metres (m^{-1}) and is designated by the letter *R*.

$$R = \frac{1}{r}$$

e.g. A lens with a radius of curvature +5*cm* [Note the importance of always stating the sign, even when it is positive] will have a curvature of:

$$R = \frac{1}{+0.05} = +20m^{-1}$$

Plus and Minus Lenses

A plus lens [otherwise known as a positive or converging lens] is one which causes parallel light to converge to a real focus. A minus lens [negative or diverging] is one which causes parallel light to diverge from a virtual focus. The effect this has on a parallel pencil of rays not only determines whether it is a plus or minus but also provides us with a means of specifying its power.

If a parallel pencil of light passes along the optical axis of a plus lens it converges to a point ***F´*** on the optical axis known as the *second principal focus*. If however the pencil passes through a minus lens it spreads out or diverges and appears to have emanated from a point ***F´*** on the optical axis, in front of the lens. [see Fig.3.8].

Lens Power

Fig.3.8

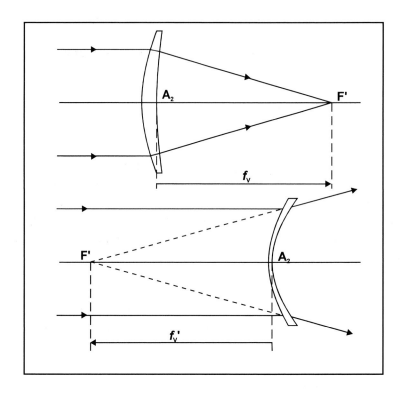

The measure of a lens to affect the curvature of incident wave-fronts is referred to as its *focal power*. Units of focal power are called dioptres and are related to the focal length (*f* or *f'*) of the lens. The focal power is symbolised by *F*, and the relationship between the focal length and focal power is expressed by the formula:

$$F = \frac{n}{f\,(metres)} = \frac{n'}{f'}$$

where *n* is the refractive index of the medium in which the light is travelling.

Light travels faster through some media than through others. It also varies with the wave-length of the light concerned. At the blue end of the visible spectrum a medium could have a refractive index of 1.530 decreasing to 1.520 at the red end of the spectrum. By tradition we use the mean refractive index for most purposes unless stated otherwise. The value we place on this mean figure is that for light in the yellow part of the spectrum. The actual number for the refractive index of a medium is obtained by comparing the speed of light in air to the speed of light in that medium [strictly speaking the comparison is between the speed in a vacuum to that in the medium which results in the *absolute refractive index*].

$$\text{Refractive index } n = \frac{\text{Velocity of light in air}}{\text{Velocity of light in medium}}$$

The total power of a thin lens is made up of the combined powers of its surfaces:

$$F = F_1 + F_2$$

The *surface power* is dependent upon the radius of curvature (r) and the mean refractive index (n) of the lens medium:

$$F_1 = \frac{n'-n}{r_1} \text{ and } F_2 = \frac{n-n'}{r_2}$$

where F_1 and F_2 are the surface powers of the first and second surface expressed in dioptres, n is the refractive index of the medium surrounding the lens [usually air ($n = 1$)], n' is the refractive index of the lens medium, and r_1 and r_2 are the radii of curvature of the respective surfaces. If the lens becomes thick then this thickness has to be taken into consideration when calculating the total lens power. However this will be discussed at a later stage.

If we consider a thin glass lens of refractive index 1.523 and a plastics lens of refractive index 1.490 both in air of refractive index 1.000, made up with one surface plane and the other with a radius of +8.72cm, then from the above formulae we have:

$$F_{1g} = \frac{1.523 - 1}{0.872} = +6.00D$$

and

$$F_{1p} = \frac{1.490 - 1}{0.872} = +5.62D$$

thus demonstrating the effect of a change in the refractive index of the medium.

The surface power for the second surface can be calculated in the same way using the formula for F_2. Then if the lens is considered to be thin the total power of the lens can be found by adding the two surface powers together ($F = F_1 + F_2$). Where thick lenses are involved, as mentioned previously, then the thickness must be taken into consideration as it will affect the total power of the lens. We will consider thick lenses at a later stage.

The lens measure

The power of a lens surface may be found with a fair degree of accuracy with an instrument known as a **lens measure.** This is a simple form of three-legged spherometer, the legs being of circular cross-section with the ends tapering off to virtual points. Only the middle leg is movable, the outer pair marking off, in effect , a chord of predetermined length **2y** (Fig.3.9). The middle leg is spring-loaded so that a three-point contact can be maintained on the steepest concave surface within the range of the instrument. As shown in the diagram what the instrument does is to measure the sag **s** corresponding to a fixed semi-aperture **y**, the dial being calibrated so as to record the result directly in terms of surface power. This can refer to one selected refractive index, normally 1.523 (see also Appendix 2).

Fig.3.9

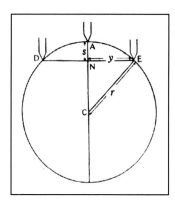

Fig.3.10 Optician's lens measure

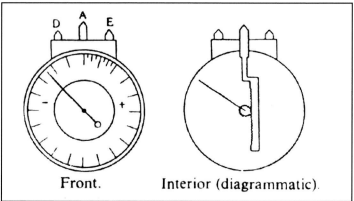

From Fig.3.11 and Fig.3.12 we can see how the lens thicknesses of different lens forms are calculated using the following rules:

bi-convex	$t = s_1 + s_2 + e,$	$e = t - [s_1 + s_2]$
plano-convex	$t = s + e,$	$e = t - s$
positive meniscus	$t = s_1 - s_2 + e,$	$e = t - [s_1 - s_2]$
bi-concave	$e = s_1 + s_2 + t,$	$t = e - [s_1 + s_2]$
plano-concave	$e = s + t,$	$t = e - s$
negative meniscus	$e = s_2 + t - s_1$	$t = e + s_1 - s_2 \, .$

Fig.3.11   Thickness of positive lenses

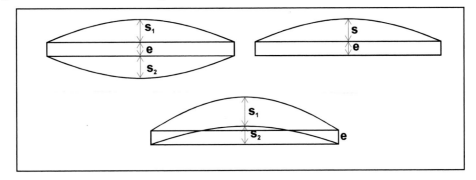

Fig.3.12   Thickness of negative lenses

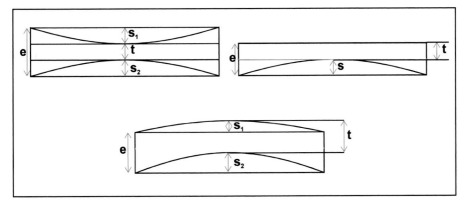

Examples:

(1) Calculate the centre thickness of a plano-convex lens made in spectacle crown glass (n = 1 523). The power of the convex surface is + 10.00DS, the diameter of the lens 40*mm* and the edge substance 1*mm*.

The radius of curvature of the curved surface must first be found from

$$r = \frac{(n-1)}{F}$$

$$r = \frac{0.523}{10} = 0.0523m$$

The semi-aperture of the lens *y* = 0.02*m*,

thus $s = 0.523 - \sqrt{[0.523^2 - 0.02^2]} = 0.0398m = 3.98mm.$

The centre thickness $t = s + e = 4.98mm$.   When a lens has two curved surfaces, the sum or difference of the sags must be calculated i.e. the formula must be applied twice.

(2) Calculate the edge substance of a −10.00DS meniscus lens, made in spectacle crown glass, the surface powers of which are +4.00DS and −14.00DS. The lens is 44*mm* in diameter and has a central thickness of 0.6*mm*.

We have $t = 0.6mm$ $F_1 = +4.00D$

$y = 22mm$ $F_2 = -14.00D.$

Proceeding as before, $r_1 = \dfrac{0.523}{4} = 0.1308m$

$r_2 = \dfrac{-0.523}{-14} = 0.03736m$

and

$s_1 = 0.1308 - \sqrt{[0.1308^2 - 0.022^2]} = 0.00186m$

$s_2 = 0.0376 - \sqrt{[0.0376^2 - 0.022^2]} = 0.00717m$

Since $e = s_2 - s_1 + t = 0.00717 - 0.00186 + 0.0006,$

the edge thickness, $e = 0.00591m = 5.91mm.$

Vergences

I am sure that all of you have, at some stage in your life, tried to set fire to grass or a piece of paper using a magnifying lens, thus demonstrating the principle that rays from a distant source [i.e. parallel] will be brought to a focus by a plus or converging lens, at the focal length of that lens.

With spectacle lenses we often have to consider rays of light which are not parallel and, as such, will therefore not come to a focus at the focal point of the lens but at some other point. That point may be calculated by the use of the formula:

$$\frac{n}{\ell} = L \quad \text{and} \quad \frac{n'}{\ell'} = L'$$

where n and n' represent the refractive indices of the media and ℓ the distance of the object or ℓ' the *image point from the lens*. L and L' are used for the vergence when measured to the object and image respectively and are measured in Dioptres.

If the object and image are in air then the formulae simplify to:

$$\frac{1}{\ell} = L \quad \text{and} \quad \frac{1}{\ell'} = L'$$

The relationship between the entering and leaving vergences can be expressed as:

$$L + F = L' \text{ or more commonly } F = L' - L$$

Parallel rays have a vergence of zero, therefore if we consider parallel light entering a $+10D$ lens we can calculate the vergence of the light leaving the lens from $L + F = L'$.

$$\ell = \infty \therefore L = \frac{1}{\infty} = 0$$

$$0.00 + (10.00) = L'$$

$$\therefore L' = \frac{1}{\ell'} \text{ where } \ell' = \frac{1}{10} = 0.1m = 10cm$$

which is equivalent to the focal length of the lens.

If we now consider light from a point $50cm$ to the left of the same lens [It is normal practice to consider light travelling from left to right, but this will be covered later] then we get the situation illustrated in Fig.3.13.

Fig.3.13

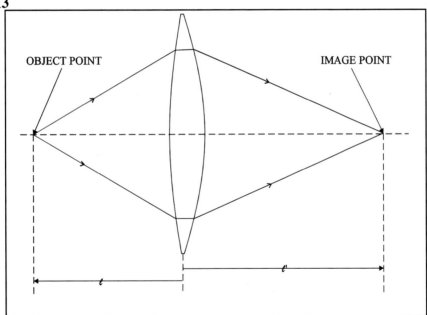

OBJECT POINT

IMAGE POINT

As ℓ and ℓ' are measured from the lens, $\ell = -0.50m$, therefore:

$$L = \frac{1}{-0.50} = -2.00D$$

$$L + F = L'$$

$$\therefore -2.00 + (+10.00) = L'$$

$$\therefore L' = +8.00D \text{ and } \ell' = \frac{1}{+8.00} = +0.125m = +12.5cm$$

We can see therefore that light leaving a point object $50cm$ from a plus lens diverges until it reaches the lens and is then converged to a focus $12.5cm$ to the right of the lens.

If we replace the $+10.00D$ lens with a $-10.00D$ lens [Fig.3.10] then the calculation is as follows:

$$L = -2.00D \text{ as before}$$

$$\therefore -2.00 + (-10.00) = L'$$

$$\therefore L' = -12.00D \text{ and } l' = \frac{1}{-12.00} = -0.83m = -8.3cm$$

In other words light leaves the negative lens as if coming from a point $8.3cm$ to the left of the lens.

Fig.3.14

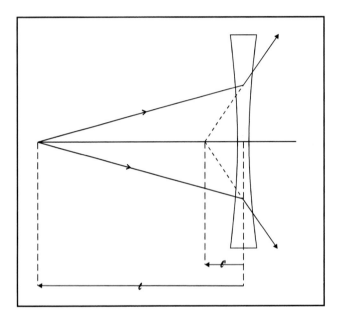

Refraction by a Lens

The change in direction of any ray on passing through a lens may be found by considering the refraction at each surface in turn. This may either be calculated from the law of refraction or may be found graphically by one of the methods previously described. It will be noticed that pencils of light on emerging from the lens are no longer homocentric. As will be expected from the result of refractions at a single curved surface, there will be spherical aberration, the rays through the more peripheral portions of the lens crossing the optical axis closer to the lens than the rays from the more central portions of the lens aperture.

Rays close to the optical axis, that is, in the paraxial region, meet the axis after refraction approximately in one point, and we shall assume that for the paraxial region point images are formed of point objects.

Focal Power

The function of the lens is to change the vergence of the light or the curvature of the wave fronts, thus producing an image - real or virtual - of the object from which the light is coming. This change in reduced vergence that the lens produces is termed its focal power. As this depends, in the case of a thin lens, only on the curvature of the surfaces and the refractive indices, the focal power of any one lens is a constant. The expressions obtained for the focal power of a surface may be applied to each surface of the lens in turn, and we have for the paraxial region

First surface.

$$\frac{n'_1}{\ell'_1} - \frac{n_1}{\ell_1} = \frac{n'_1 - n_1}{r_1}$$

Second surface

$$\frac{n'_2}{\ell'_2} - \frac{n_2}{\ell_2} = \frac{n'_2 - n_2}{r_2}$$

$$n_2 = n''_1$$

If the thickness of the lens is neglected, the vergence $\dfrac{1}{\ell'_1}$, of the refracted light at the first surface is the vergence $\dfrac{1}{\ell_2}$ of the incident light at the second surface, and

$\dfrac{n_2}{\ell_2} = \dfrac{n'_1}{\ell'_1}$ Then from the expressions above for the separate surfaces

$$\frac{n'_2}{\ell'_2} - \frac{n'_1}{\ell'_1} = \frac{n'_1 - n_1}{r_1} + \frac{n'_2 - n_2}{r_2}$$

As $\dfrac{n'_2}{\ell'_2}$ and $\dfrac{n_1}{\ell_1}$ are the reduced vergences of the incident and emergent light respectively, the expression gives the focal power of a thin lens with media of any refractive index in the object and image spaces.

Thin lens in air

If the lens is in air, then $n_1 = n'_2 = 1$ and putting

$$n'_1 = n_2 = n \quad \text{we have}$$

$$\frac{1}{\ell'_2} - \frac{1}{\ell_1} = \frac{n-1}{r_1} + \frac{1-n}{r_2} = F_1 + F_2$$

where F_1 and F_2 are the surface powers.

$$\frac{1}{\ell'_2} - \frac{1}{\ell_1} = (n-1)\left(\frac{1}{r_1} - \frac{1}{r_2}\right)$$

or, dropping the suffixes of ℓ'_2 and ℓ_1

$$\frac{1}{\ell'} - \frac{1}{\ell} = (n-1)\left(\frac{1}{r_1} - \frac{1}{r_2}\right) = L' - L \quad .. \qquad .. \qquad [3.01]$$

$L' - L$ is the focal power, F, of the lens and we have

$$F = (n-1)\left(\frac{1}{r_1} - \frac{1}{r_2}\right) = (n-1)(R_1 - R_2) \quad .. \qquad [3.02]$$

or
$$\left.\begin{array}{r} F = L' - L \\ L' = L + F \end{array}\right\} \quad .. \qquad .. \qquad .. \qquad .. \qquad [3.03]$$

For a lens in air L and L' are the vergences at the lens of the incident and emergent light respectively, and the expression [3.03] may be stated as follows:

For a lens in air, the final vergence L' of the light is equal to the incident vergence L plus the impressed vergence F.

4. ASTIGMATIC LENSES

A spherical surface is equally curved in all meridians and so the surface curvature of a spherical lens duplicates the surface curvature of a sphere. If however we now consider surfaces other than spherical ones, there is another important type of spectacle lens which is referred to as *astigmatic*.

The simplest form of astigmatic lens is one that is formed by a section of a cylinder [Fig.4.1]

Fig.4.1

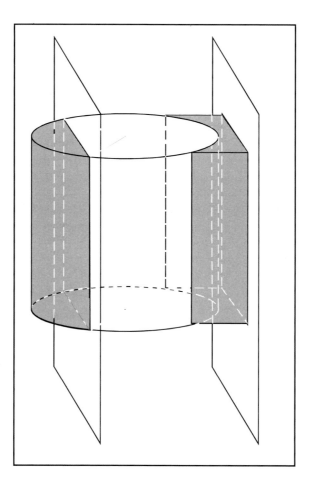

Because a cylinder can be turned from a vertical to a horizontal position, or for that matter any position in between, we must choose a method of specifying its exact orientation when talking about cylindrical lenses.

In Fig.4.1 the line YY´ is the *axis of revolution* of the cylinder. Any line on the surface of the surface of the cylinder which is parallel to this line is known as the *axis meridian*. The directions at right angles to this meridian are *power meridians*.

A cylindrical lens can be used to correct an eye that does not bring rays of light to a point focus. One reason for this could be that the cornea is more curved in one meridian than in another. A cylindrical lens is suited for correcting this error because light that strikes the lens along the axis of the lens will pass through it undeviated, whereas light which strikes it at right angles to the axis [power meridian] will be refracted according to the power of the lens in this meridian. [Fig.4.2]. The power of a cylindrical lens is also stated in Dioptres and is usually designated the symbol DC to differentiate it from DS [Dioptre Sphere].

Fig.4.2

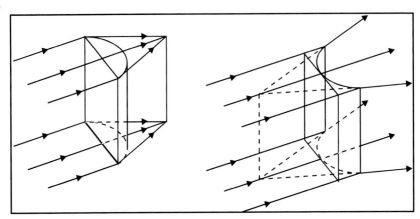

Sphero-cylindrical lenses

As stated previously a cylindrical lens is used to correct an astigmatic eye that does not bring light to a single point focus. Unfortunately astigmatism doesn't often occur in isolation but more frequently in combination with *myopia* [short-sightedness] or *hyperopia* [long-sightedness]. Therefore it becomes necessary to correct the subject's refractive defect by the use of both spherical and cylindrical lenses. the resulting combination is referred to as a *sphero-cylindrical lens.*

Light passing through a sphero-cylindrical lens combination would be refracted as shown in Fig.4.3 which illustrates a positive sphere combined with a positive cylinder.

To write the power and orientation characteristics of a sphero-cylindrical lens we have to include three elements - *sphere* or *spherical power - cylindrical power* and *cylinder axis.*

Fig.4.3

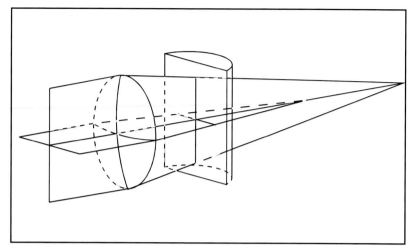

If the spherical part of the combination were to be +5.00*DS* and the cylindrical element +3.00*DC* at an axis of 90°, the lens combination is usually written as:

+5.00*DS*/+3.00*DC* ax 90

All sphero-cylindrical lenses have two different power meridians. Along the axis meridian of a cylindrical surface it is flat and hence has zero power or if it is combined with a spherical surface then the power is that of the sphere alone. In the other principal meridian the cylinder contributes to the total power of the lens [Fig.4.4]. Remember that the power meridian is at right angles to the axis meridian.

Fig.4.4

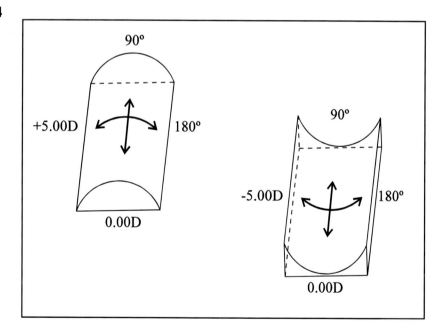

We must add together the sphere power and the cylinder power in order to obtain the total combined power in the respective principal meridians. If we consider the lens with the power of +5.00DS/+3.00DC axis 90 then it will have a power of +5.00D vertically and +8.00D horizontally.

Transposition

It can now be shown that an astigmatic lens of specified principal powers can be made up in two different sphero-cylindrical forms. Let us suppose we require a lens with principal powers as follows:

+2.00D along the 60° meridian and
+5.00D along the 150° meridian.

We could of course use a +2.00D sphere and combine it with a +3.00D cylinder with its axis at 60°.

Alternatively we could use a +5.00D sphere and combine it with a –3.00D cylinder with its axis at 150°.

If we express the lens combinations in the conventional manner we get:

1.   +2.00DS/+3.00DC axis 60
2.   +5.00DS/–3.00DC axis 150

The two prescriptions above for the same lens are termed alternative transpositions. The word transposition is also used for the process of converting from one form to another without a change of lens power.

Rules of transposition

Transposition can be carried out by the use of the following simple rules:

1.   Add the sphere and cylinder values to obtain the new sphere value.
2.   Change the sign of the cylinder [plus to minus or minus to plus].
3.   Change the axis by 90° [This can be done by adding 90° if the original was less than 90° or if the original was over 90° then subtract 90° from it].

E.g.   (a) +2.50DS/+0.75DC ax 30
             becomes
             +3.25DS/–0.75DC ax 120   (c) +2.00DS/–4.00DC ax 60
                                                            becomes
         (b) –2.00DS/+2.00DC ax 45   –2.00DS/+4.00DC ax 150
             becomes
             Plano/–2.00DC ax 135

5. TORIC LENSES

Lenses can be made in a variety of forms, with many forms possible for a lens of the same power. A lens of a specified power can for example be made with a cylinder component on the back or front surface. One lens may be steeply curved, whilst another, of identical power, may appear flatter.

If you remember when we considered astigmatic lenses and sphero-cylindrical lens combinations we had one surface spherical in form and the other was cylindrical. We are now going to look at lenses which have one surface spherical but the other having a sphere and a cylinder combined together. This is known as a *toroidal* surface.

A toroidal surface is generated by rotating the arc of a circle DAD' about an axis of revolution OO' which lies in the same plane as the arc but does not pass through its centre of curvature C [Fig.5.1].

Fig.5.1

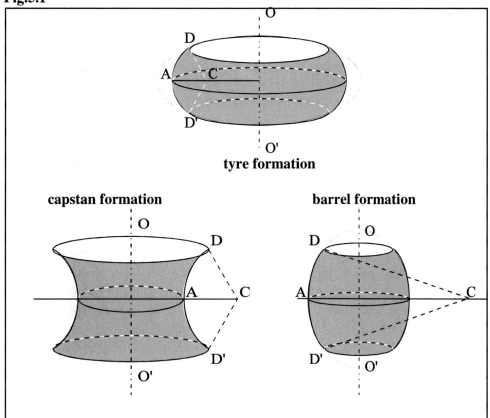

tyre formation

capstan formation

barrel formation

If the axis of revolution OO' lies on the side of C remote from the vertex A of the arc, then the toroidal surface takes on a *tyre formation*. If however OO' lies between A and C the resulting surface is of the *barrel formation*. The third possibility is where OO' and C lie on opposite sides of A giving rise to the *capstan formation*.

With a toroidal surface the meridian with the least curvature is called the *base curve*. It follows that the meridian with the greatest power, which is always at right angles to the base curve, is called the *cross curve*. A convex toroidal surface is called a *plus base toric* and a concave surface is called a *minus base toric*. The surface on the opposite side of the lens to the toroidal surface is logically called the *sphere curve*.

Toric lenses

Toric lenses have one surface which is convex and one which is concave, either of which is toroidal.

Fig.5.2

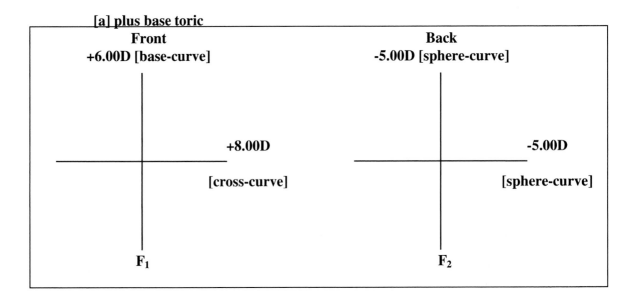

[a] plus base toric

Front	Back
+6.00D [base-curve]	-5.00D [sphere-curve]
+8.00D	-5.00D
[cross-curve]	[sphere-curve]
F₁	F₂

[b] minus base toric

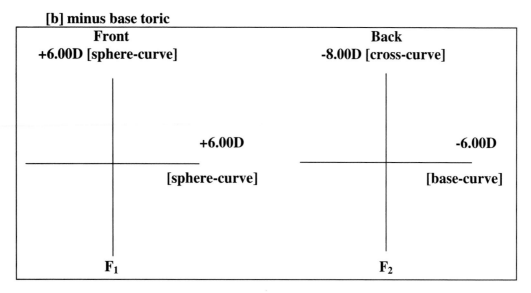

As before the nominal power of a lens $F_T = F_1 + F_2$, therefore in the examples above [a] has nominal powers of +1.00D in the vertical meridian and +3.00D in the horizontal meridian and could be represented by the sphero-cylindrical form +1.00DS/+2.00DC ax 90. [b] has nominal powers of –2.00D in the vertical meridian and 0.00D in the horizontal meridian and is represented by Plano/–2.00DC ax 180.

Both of these lenses could be represented in their toric transposition form:

[a] $$\frac{+6.00DC\times180/+8.00DC\times90}{-5.00DS}$$

[b] $$\frac{+6.00DS}{-6.00DC\times90/-8.00DC\times180}$$

It should be fairly easy to see from the above that if two spheres are placed together a new sphere is the result. If a sphere and a cylinder are placed together then a sphero-cylinder results. However if we place two equal cylinders together but with their axes at right angles to one another then a sphere results [Fig.5.3]. If the cylinders are not equal then a sphero-cylinder results.

Note that when writing prescriptions the **ax** is often replaced by just ×. See Fig.5.3 on the next page.

Fig.5.3

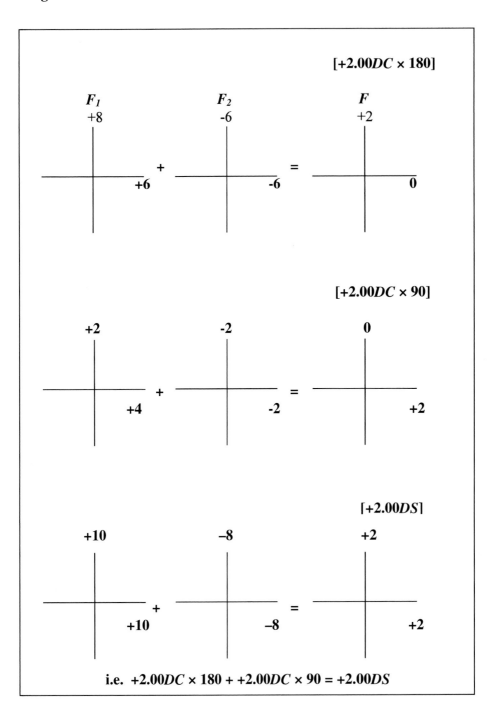

i.e. $+2.00DC \times 180 + +2.00DC \times 90 = +2.00DS$

6. BEST FORM LENSES

An ideal lens would reunite all the rays emanating from each point on the object and bring them to a focus at the corresponding point on the image. The image would also be an exact-to-scale reproduction of the object.

In actual fact, a simple lens does not behave in this way but is subject to various *aberrations* that impair the quality of the image. Although a detailed study of lens aberrations demands advanced mathematics, their effects may be summarised quite simply: they are loss of definition [blurring], distortion [for example straight lines appear curved] and chromatism [colour fringes]. Each of these defects may be observed on viewing some fine print through a strong magnifying lens. Towards the edges of the field of view there will generally be a marked deterioration in the quality of the image.

Spectacle lenses are subject to similar aberrations, which the wearer may notice, especially when looking through them obliquely. The amount of each aberration depends not only on the power of the lens but also on the form in which it is made.

A great deal of study and calculation has been devoted to the problem of determining the theoretically best base curve for every lens power. Unfortunately in the field of optical design, it is seldom possible to achieve one's aims entirely. The base curve required to eliminate one aberration may not deal successfully with others. There are also differences of opinion as to which aberration is the most objectionable and hence should be given prior consideration. Since the beginning of the century, a number of lens computers in different countries have formulated various requirements as the ideal and have worked out the base curves which lenses should have in order to satisfy this ideal.

Unfortunately when designing lens forms to eliminate or reduce the various aberrations, certain 'average' parameters have to be assumed, such as the distance the lens will sit in front of the eye and the distance the front of the eye is from the centre of its rotation. However one has to start somewhere and a series of lenses produced in accordance with such a scheme is generally termed *best-form*.

A best form lens is one which is designed to minimise the effects of oblique astigmatism and therefore provides the best vision for objects viewed obliquely. Secondary considerations are distortion and transverse chromatic aberration, although only a little control of these is possible, if at all.

In recent years, analysis of lens form has been revolutionised by the advent of the personal computer. The possibility of rapidly calculating spectacle lens performance is now a reality. Calculations which took hours to do in the past can now be done in seconds. This allows us to examine lens performance by comparing the results of exact ray tracing in the oblique gaze positions. As an example of the influence of form, consider a +6.00DS lens in three forms, each with the eye rotated 30°, the eye's centre of rotation 27mm from the back vertex of the lens, the refractive index of the lens 1.523 and the V-number 59. The oblique powers are shown in Table 6.1 in sph/cyl form, together with the distortion and the chromatic aberration:

Table 6.1   Various forms of a +6.00DS lens. Uncut diameter 60mm, with edge thickness 2mm, ocular rotation 30° and fitting distance 27mm. n = 1.523.

Back surface power	Oblique power	Distortion	Transverse Chromatic Aberration[TCA]	Centre thickness
0.00	+6.22DS/+1.37DC	8.92%	0.20 Δ	6.68 mm
−3.75	+5.83DS/+0.36DC	6.26%	0.19 Δ	6.94 mm
−7.12	+5.65DS/ 0.00DC	4.76%	0.19 Δ	7.51 mm

This example illustrates that form has a significant effect on oblique gaze focus. We refer to the details as the oblique performance of the lens. Opticians should understand these effects and whenever necessary should dispense spectacles with best-form theory in mind.

The origin of oblique astigmatism

Oblique astigmatism arises because of the asymmetry in the refraction of the rays in two mutually perpendicular planes - the tangential and sagittal planes. These planes are illustrated in Fig.6.2. Note that a meridional ray is one which, produced if necessary, intersects the principal axis.

Tangential plane - is one which includes the meridional ray and the principal axis of the surface.

Sagittal plane - is that plane which is perpendicular to the tangential plane and includes the meridional ray.

In Fig.6.2, these planes intersect the surface in the tangential and sagittal meridians, labelled **T** and **S** in the diagram. It is the angles of incidence which differ and thereby introduce the asymmetrical refraction which produces oblique astigmatism. Fig.6.3 shows how the angles of incidence in the tangential and sagittal planes differ at the points **A, B, D** and **E.**

Fig.6.2 The tangential and sagittal meridians T and S. P_T' and P_S' are the tangential and sagittal line foci. D is the disc of least confusion.

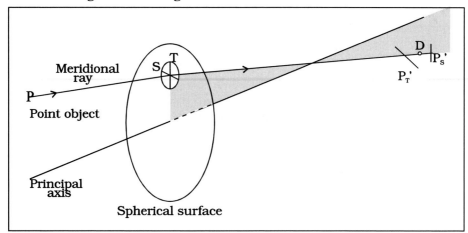

Fig.6.3 [a]The angles of incidence in the tangential meridian AB: $i_A = i_B$
[b]The angles of incidence in the sagittal meridian DE: $i_D = i_E$ C is the centre of curvature of the surface and the dashed lines are normals at the points A, B, D and E.

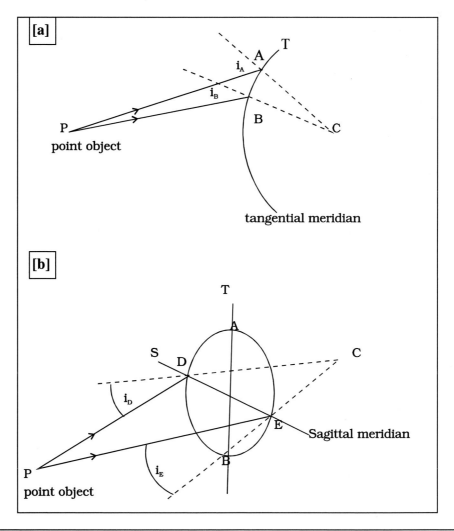

Calculation of oblique astigmatism

Coddington's equations are used to calculate the positions of the line foci. In these equations, quoted below, *t* and *s* are the object distances which are equal at the first surface of a system since the light originates from the point object on the meridional ray. The image distances for the tangential and sagittal line foci are *t'* and *s'*. The angles of incidence and refraction for the meridional ray are *i* and *i'*, respectively. Note that the rays in Fig.6.3[a] and [b] are to be imagined as straddling the meridional ray and they are infinitesimally close to it. This is similar to the situation with the more familiar paraxial ray theory and a meridional ray can therefore be considered as a secondary axis.

Coddington's equations

In the sagittal plane

$$\frac{n'}{s'} - \frac{n}{s} = \frac{n'.\cos i' - n.\cos i}{r}$$

In the tangential plane

$$\frac{n'.\cos^2 i'}{t'} - \frac{n.\cos^2 i}{t} = \frac{n'.\cos i' - n.\cos i}{r}$$

The right hand side of each equation is called the *oblique astigmatic power*. As a matter of interest, note the effect of small *i* and *i'*: this leads to the paraxial equation in both cases; i.e.

$$\frac{n'}{\ell'} - \frac{n}{\ell} = \frac{n'-n}{r}$$

where the ℓ symbol replaces the *s* and *t* symbols and the point object on the axis.

Fig.6.4 **Illustration of the tangential and sagittal object and image distances for oblique refraction at a spherical surface.**

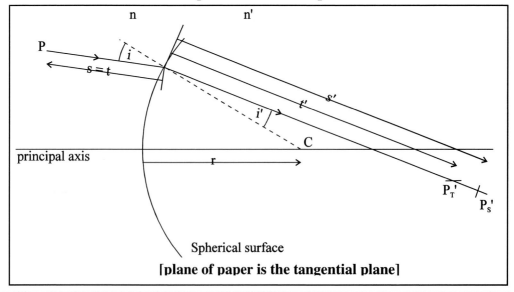

[plane of paper is the tangential plane]

Coddington's equations applied to a spectacle lens

Here the eye's centre of rotation **R** is a fixed point behind and on the principal axis of the lens. This is a design criterion which should be remembered since it will be shown to have much practical importance in dispensing.

Fig.6.5 shows the familiar paraxial treatment of a lens correcting a hypermetropic eye. Rays from a distant axial point are focused at the eye's far point M_R. Note the distance from the spectacle point S to the far point M_R is equal to the back vertex focal length $f_v{}'$ of the lens.

In Fig.6.6, the eye is shown rotated through an angle $U_2{}'$ which may be called the ocular rotation or the slope angle of the emergent ray. The ray through the centre of the eye's pupil [not shown] is the chief ray or meridional ray.

An exact ray trace commences by stating the value of $U_2{}'$, say 30°, stating the fitting distance **SR** [say 27*mm*], then tracing the ray backwards into object space. During this stage the angles of incidence and refraction at the surfaces are calculated. The object point is then stated to be at infinity or some near position on this chief ray, after which Coddington's equations are used to find the positions of the line foci by forward refraction at the two spectacle lens surfaces. The distance δ of the ray in the lens is calculated from the x and y co-ordinates of the points M and N which are themselves calculated from the geometry.

Fig.6.5   **The familiar correction of hypermetropia with an axial point object at infinity. M_R is the eye's far point, S is the spectacle point, and R is the eye's centre of rotation.**

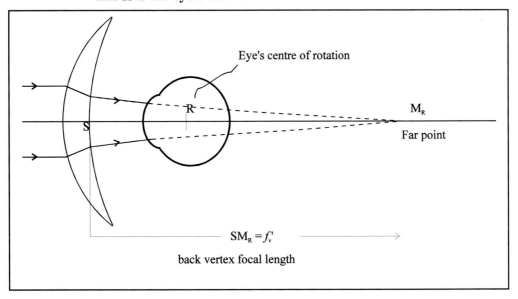

Fig.6.6   **Some of the detail involved in the calculation of the positions of the tangential and sagittal line foci.**

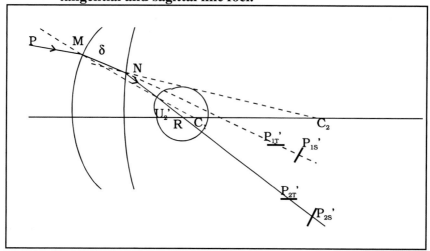

$MN = \delta$ = distance in the lens
$MP_{1T}' = t_1'$
$MP_{1S}' = s_1'$
$NP_{2T}' = t_2'$
$NP_{2S}' = s_2'$
    $s_2 = s_1' - \delta$
    $t_2 = t_1' - \delta$

Best form lens terminology

Fig.6.7 will be used to introduce the terminology involved in best form lens design for distance vision. Two important concepts are apparent in this figure; the *Far Point Sphere* and the *Vertex Sphere*. These are formed by rotating the far point M_R and the spectacle point S about the eye's centre of rotation R. Of course, only arcs are shown here but you can imagine each one as part of their respective spheres. The object is a distant point on the chief [meridional] ray, so the tangential and sagittal line foci are labelled F_T' and F_S' respectively. The disc of least confusion is marked D.

Note that the focal lengths f_T' and f_S' are measured from the Vertex Sphere. The reason for this is so that dioptric quantities such as the Mean Oblique Power can be compared directly with the back vertex power of the lens; i.e. the dioptric equivalents of all image distances can then be compared directly with the Back Vertex Power $F_v' = 1/f_v'$ of the lens. The various terms are introduced as follows;

Best form lens terminology for a distance vision lens

f_T' is the tangential oblique vertex sphere focal length.
    It is the distance QF_T'
f_s' is the sagittal oblique vertex sphere focal length.
    It is the distance QF_S'
$F_T = 1/f_T'$ is the tangential oblique vertex sphere power [TOVSP].
$F_S = 1/f_S'$ is the sagittal oblique vertex sphere power [SOVSP].

The oblique astigmatic error [OAE] is then simply:

$$OAE = F_T - F_S$$

The dioptric distance of the disc of least confusion from the far point sphere. This is given by $\frac{1}{2}[F_T + F_S]$ and is known as the Mean Oblique Power [MOP]. That is:

$$MOP = \frac{1}{2}[F_T + F_S]$$

The amount by which the MOP differs from the back vertex power of the lens $[F_v{'}]$ is known as the Mean Oblique Error [MOE], so that:

$$MOE = MOP - F_v{'}$$

Another important term is the Tangential Error [TE]. This is the amount by which the Tangential Oblique Vertex Power F_T differs from the back vertex of the lens i.e.:

$$TE = F_T - F_v{'}$$

Fig.6.7 **Illustrating the Far Point Sphere and the Vertex Sphere.**

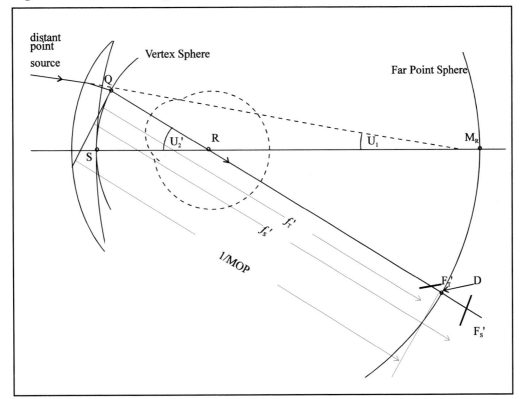

Ideal best form lens

**Fig 6.8   Illustration of the ideal best form lens in which a point focus forms
on the far point sphere in oblique gaze. Thus OAE = 0 and MOE = 0.**

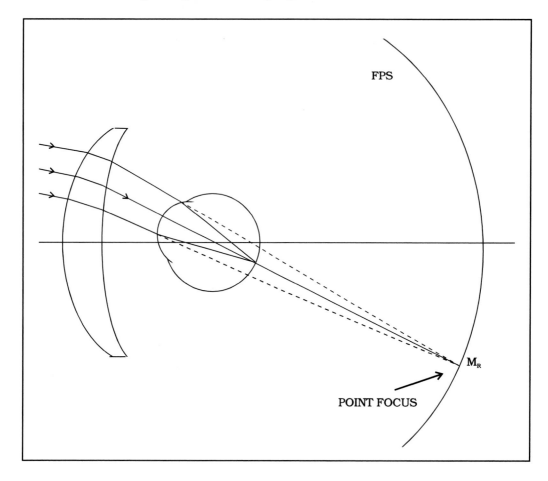

7. ASPHERIC LENSES

As you may remember from Chapter 2 the dispensing of lenses was a comparatively simple matter in 'the old days'. Uncut single vision lenses were flat 55Ø round. Ultimately lenses became curved and larger - meniscus in 60Ø, 65Ø, 70Ø and even 80Ø. Along with what seemed at the time like a revolution, but was I suspect only evolution, we 'discovered' aberrations such as oblique astigmatism and mean oblique error. Obviously we didn't really discover these problems but the means to improve upon the solutions were becoming more apparent and available as well as viable.

The most serious problem to be overcome with spectacle lens design is that of oblique astigmatism. If you reconsider the previous chapter you will see that oblique astigmatism can be reduced or eliminated altogether by 'bending' the lens. Unfortunately this often results in lenses with a bulbous appearance which is cosmetically unacceptable.

A 'best form' lens will also inevitably produce what is known as mean oblique error which is expressed in dioptres as the average power at a certain angle away from the optical centre compared with the power at the optical centre.

In order to solve the problem of bulbous lenses and therefore provide thinner and flatter lenses and yet still retain lenses which are relatively free from oblique astigmatism and mean oblique error, lens manufacturers have utilised computers and computer controlled machinery to produce aspherical surfaces.

As long ago as the early 1900's Ernst Abbe, and Moritz von Rohr described aspheric lenses and Zeiss produced a version under the name of Katral. Variations on a theme took place over the years but it wasn't until the 60's and the arrival of CR39 on the scene that any significant advances took place. Many of these lenses were being produced for the correction of aphakia. In 1980 Mo Jalie patented a design for low power aspherics with the aspheric surface on the front for plus lenses and the aspheric surface on the back of a minus lens. However lenses are currently manufactured with the aspheric surface on the convex side irrespective of whether they are plus or minus.

Strictly speaking we could call any surface which is not spherical an aspherical one but we reserve this term for an optical surface which has rotational but non-circular symmetry about its optical axis. In this context we can call upon the other members of the conicoid family to which the circle also belongs. These curved forms get their name from the fact that they are all sections of a cone as shown in Fig.7.1. Their mathematical derivations from the formula: $y^2 = 2r_0x - px^2$ are shown in Fig.7.2. They are an oblate ellipse, circle, prolate ellipse, parabola and hyperbola where the type of curve is determined by the value given to p.

e.g. Where the value of $p>1$ then the curve is an oblate ellipse.   [imaginary]

   "   "   "   " $p=1$ "   "   "   " a circle.

   "   "   "   " $p<1$ but>0 "   "   " a prolate ellipse.

   "   "   "   " $p=0$ then "   "   " a parabola.

   "   "   "   " $p<o$ "   "   "   " a hyperbola.

Fig.7.1 Sections of a Cone

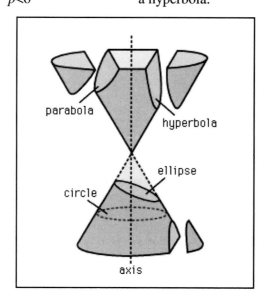

Fig.7.2 The Conicoid Family

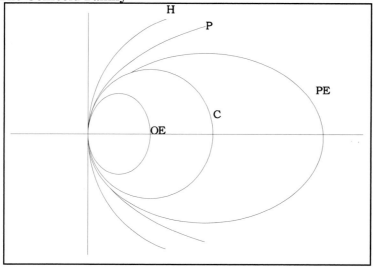

The purpose of using an aspherical surface is to introduce negative surface astigmatism which effectively neutralises the oblique astigmatism. Because these surfaces have smaller sags than their spherical counterparts there is also a reduction in thickness.

The rate at which a hyperbolic surface flattens is such that it is right for introducing this negative surface astigmatism and therefore ideal for neutralising the oblique astigmatism which would have been produced by a spherical surface.

If a high refractive index material is used in the manufacture of these aspherical surfaces then a further considerable saving in thickness is effected.

8. NEUTRALISATION/FOCIMETER

Eutralisation, or hand neutralisation as it is known, is a relatively simple and accurate method of determining the power of an unknown lens. The only equipment that is required is a set of lenses such as those available in any trial set, and a crossline chart. A crossline chart can easily be constructed by drawing two lines at right angles to one another on a piece of stiff paper or card. The cross bars of a window or door panel can also be utilised.

The object of the exercise is to determine the power of the unknown lens by placing in contact with it a lens or series of known lenses of equal but opposite power so that the net result of the combination is zero power. The unknown lens is then said to be neutralised.

The method of neutralisation in this way is essentially one of trial and error, but practice and experience can lead to fast and accurate results. As with all experimental work when determining an unknown we must apply a series of tests and from the results of these tests decide what is indicated. Negative results are as important as positive ones. When neutralising lenses therefore we must apply the tests relating to astigmatic lenses as well as those for spherical lenses and only when a negative result is obtained is it safe to assume that a lens is spherical and not astigmatic.

Transverse movements

If we view a crossline chart or similar object through a piece of plane glass and then move the glass from side to side and then up and down in directions which are parallel to the lines of the crossline chart we will perceive no apparent movement of the lines. However if the experiment is repeated with a minus spherical lens instead of the plane glass, then it will be seen that the lines of the chart appear to move in the same direction as the direction of movement of the minus lens. This is known as a with movement.

Repeating the exercise with a plus lens instead of a minus lens will result in the crosslines appearing to move in the opposite direction to that of the lens and is known as an against movement. If a high-powered plus lens is held sufficiently far away from the observer's eye then an apparent with movement will be observed, but as it will be obvious that it is a strong plus lens, confusion should not occur. The image will also be inverted. During the process of neutralisation of a high-powered plus lens the lens combination will gradually become weaker and therefore the apparent movement will revert to an against movement.

When the stage is reached that there is no apparent movement, then neutralisation has been achieved.

Fig.8.1 Scissors movement

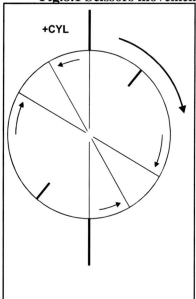

+CYL

If the major axes of an astigmatic lens are parallel to the lines of the crossline chart then by moving the lens as described above a with or against movement will be observed. Different amounts of movement or even opposite types of movement will be observed depending upon the powers of the lens along the major axes.

By observing the crossline chart through a lens and rotating it, when a spherical lens is under scrutiny, then the lines will remain unchanged. However if the lens is astigmatic then the lines will appear to rotate in different directions from one another giving rise to the term scissors movement [Fig.8.1]. At some point during the rotation test, as it is known, the crosslines as observed through the lens will be continuous with those of the chart itself. It is at this point that the major axes of the lens are in line with the chart lines, which is useful for marking the major axes on the lens.

Neutralising spherical lenses

Take the unknown lens and hold the top and bottom edges between thumb and forefinger at about arms length and by performing the transverse test, i.e., moving it from side to side or up and down and viewing the crossline chart through it, estimate the power and sign of the lens. As state previously if the lens is a plus sphere it will give an against movement and if it is a minus sphere it will give a with movement. By taking a spherical lens of known power from the trial case and placing it in the closest contact with the unknown lens and performing the transverse test again you will know from the result how close you are to neutralisation. The closest contact between the two lenses will depend upon the form of the lenses. For example if the unknown lens is a plus meniscus then the closest contact will be attained by placing the curved minus side of the trial lens in contact with the convex surface of the meniscus lens.

Let us suppose that the unknown lens is a –4.50D sphere. Firstly by holding the lens at arms length and viewing the crossline chart and performing the transverse test we will observe a with movement. If we estimate the power to be of the order of –4.00D, we take a +4.00D trial lens and place it in closest contact with the unknown lens and perform the transverse test again. This time because the combination is still negative we will perceive a with movement but not so pronounced. Suppose we decide to replace the +4.00D trial lens with a +5.00D and repeat the exercise, this time we will see an against movement because the combination is now positive. By changing the trial lens and a process of elimination we should eventually reach a situation of no movement and a zero power combination and hence neutralisation.

It may be necessary to use more than one trial lens to obtain the desired combination. Inevitably due to lens thickness and incomplete contact between the lens surfaces there will some peripheral distortion observed as well as not being able to attain complete freedom from movement. In order to reduce these problems, the following should be observed:

1. Place the crossline chart as far away as possible.
2. Hold the lenses at arms length.
3. Use the fewest number of lenses to obtain the required combination.
4. Take care to avoid scratching lenses when placed in contact with one another.
5. Remember the sign of the unknown lens is opposite to that of the trial lens(es).
6. Use a masking ring to confine observation to the central portion of the lens.

Neutralising astigmatic lenses

Exactly the same principles as the above are involved when neutralising astigmatic lenses but with additional steps. There are two methods of hand neutralising astigmatic lenses and they are as follows:

Method 1: With this method we use only spherical lenses to neutralise each of the principal meridians in turn. Firstly we carry out the rotation test which as well as confirming that the lens under consideration is astigmatic it allows us to line up the major axes with the crossline chart as described previously. The vertical meridian can now be neutralised as described for spherical lenses by moving the unknown lens, and subsequently the combination of lenses, up and down and continuing the process depending upon the results of the observations made.

The process is then repeated by observing the movements of the vertical crossline when the lens(es) are moved from side to side. The neutralisation point will give us the principal power of the lens in the horizontal meridian.

If for example the above process resulted in a +2.50D trial lens being used for the vertical meridian and a +1.00D trial lens for the horizontal meridian then the prescription can be written as:
$$-2.50DS/+1.50DC \text{ or } -1.00DS/-1.50DC.$$

The following rule may be found to be useful:

If the two principal powers are A and B then the two alternative sph-cyl forms are:
A sphere combined with (B – A) cylinder or
B sphere combined with (A – B) cylinder.
Remember to take care with signs in algebraic additions.

Method 2: As in Method 1 the unknown lens must firstly have its axes aligned with the crossline chart. A spherical trial lens is used as before to neutralise the vertical power meridian. This trial lens is retained in position whilst a second cylindrical lens is then placed in contact with the combination with its axis vertical. A series of cylindrical trial lenses is used until the neutralisation process is complete.

If for example the above process resulted in a –1.50*DS* trial lens being used for the vertical meridian and a –2.00*DC* for the horizontal meridian the resulting power of the lens under consideration would be: +1.50*DS*/+2.00*DC* or +3.50*DS*/–2.00*DC*.

As mentioned earlier due to the thickness and curvature of the unknown lens it may be found that in order to obtain close contact between it and the trial lens the front vertex power is neutralised instead of the back vertex power. There will be a significant difference between these two results with medium or high powered plus lenses. A more accurate back vertex power result can be obtained using a focimeter.

None of these methods of course tell us the form of the lens which we can determine using a lens measure.

The Focimeter

This is an instrument which is used for measuring the back vertex power of a lens as well as its orientation in a spectacle frame and also any prism or prismatic effects. Most focimeters incorporate devices for marking the centre of the lens and some have printers attached which will give a hard copy of a digital read out.

The original instrument took the form of a monocular instrument similar in appearance to a microscope. It was comprised of two parts a focusing system and an observing system. Although many embellishments have appeared over the years the principles remain unchanged in today's instruments.

The focusing system consists of a moveable target, a collimating lens and a clamping device for the lens under inspection. Because this clamping device positions the lens at the second principal focus of the collimating lens, the target always appears the same size and the movement of the target required for focusing is directly proportional to the power of the lens under test. Hence the dioptre scale is of uniform graduation.

The observing system takes the form of a telescope though which the observer views the target in order to bring it into focus. Scales indicating the power and also the axis orientation may be seen through the telescope with some instruments or viewed externally with others. As with all optical instruments of this type the eyepiece has to be set for the individual observer. If the image of the target is projected onto a screen then this is not the case and has the additional advantage that both eyes can be used together which is generally less tiring.

There are many variations on a theme available today and it is advisable for students to familiarise themselves with the setting and manipulation of as many types as possible. It should also be remembered that by turning the dials the instrument will record whatever value you stop at, whether there is a lens in the clamp or not, so do not be taken in by a print out!

Automated focimeters will automatically set the zero and take various readings of the lens under inspection when the appropriate switch is activated. Unlike the digital read out instruments mentioned previously these instruments do not require any assessment on the part of the operator

The focimeter can be divided into two parts: the focusing system, against which the test lens is clamped, and the observation system, which is a telescopic system.

Fig.8.2 A plus lens being measured by a focimeter

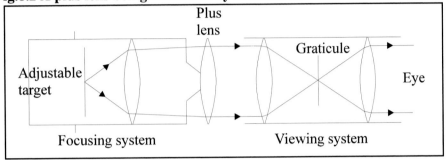

Observation system
Eyepiece

Like most optical instruments, the eyepiece can be adjusted for individual users. Indeed, it must be adjusted before use. It is recommended that you set the eyepiece by first holding a sheet of white paper between the lens stop and the telescope objective (the focimeter need not be switched on). This is similar to placing a lens for checking. Hold the paper at an angle which reflects the most light into the telescope. The lines on the graticule should be in sharp focus. If they are not, follow this procedure:

1 Turn the eyepiece anticlockwise until the lines and circles are completely blurred.
2 Turn the eyepiece clockwise until the lines are in sharp focus. If you go past the sharp focus, blur the lines again and then slowly turn back to sharp focus.
3 Switch on the focimeter's light and focus the target. The power drum should now read zero.
4 If the graticule is clear but the target is blurry when the power drum is set to zero, the instrument may need recalibrating. Recheck steps 1-3 if the target is still blurry, noting the reading on the power drum when the target is in clear focus (say, +0.50*D*). Deduct this from all the measurements you make.
For example, if the drum reads +6.50*D* the actual power is +6.00*D*. Think of it as a watch that is set 10 minutes fast—you can always tell the exact time by deducting 10 minutes.

Repeat the exercise if the power drum is not on zero.

Objective lens

The objective lens is a strong plus lens which, together with the eyepiece lens, forms an afocal system (a telescope). That is, parallel light entering the lens system will emerge parallel. The separation of the two lenses is the sum of their focal lengths.

Graticule

The graticule is a flat parallel-sided plate of glass with lines and circles etched on its surface. It is positioned at the second principal focus of the objective lens of the observation system 'telescope' (which is also the first principal focus of the eyepiece lens). By being in this position the graticule always appears to be in the same plane as the target.

The graticule is used to measure the amount and direction of prism usually up to 5Δ.

Prism cell

The prism cell is placed just behind the objective lens, between the objective lens and the lens under test. It holds auxiliary prisms to measure prisms over 5Δ These auxiliary or added prisms actually 'decentre' the centre of the target to extend the prism measurement capability of the focimeter.

They are useful if the lens you are checking or marking has ordered prism greater than the 5Δ circle which is the limit of prism marked on the graticule of most focimeters.

Your focimeter may have an inbuilt prism compensator which adjusts the centre of the target up to 15Δ, replacing the need for auxiliary prisms. It may also include the protractor, the prism dioptre scale and the vertex power scale inside the instrument. All of these are visible through the eyepiece and they speed up the measuring time.

Marking device

This device contains pins which dot the optical centre and horizontal meridian. There are three pins in a row which are pressed down into an ink tray (some focimeters have self-inking markers) before being swung up and pressed down on the lens to mark the optical centre and the horizontal meridian.

Ink well

The ink well is a container which supplies ink for the marking device (some focimeters have self-inking markers).

Clamp

The clamp holds the lens against the lens rest. It should ensure that the lens does not wobble on the lens rest. If the lens were to sit at an angle to the lens rest, it would induce cylindrical power.

Focusing system
Collimating lens

The collimating or standard lens is a strong plus lens situated just below the lens rest. Its purpose is to collimate (make parallel) the divergent light from the target. This parallel light will then pass through the observation system.

Lens rest

The lens rest is a circular aperture of about *5mm* diameter, positioned at the second principal focus of the collimating lens. By being in that position the target will always appear the same size, regardless of the power of the lens under test, and the graduations on the power drum will all be the same. The lens is held by the clamp against the lens rest. Some focimeters allow this aperture to be reduced for checking, for example progressives.

Target

The target, illuminated by a globe just beneath it, comes in two basic types: the crossed-line target and the ring-of-dots or corona target. We will look at both types and the recent hybrids that have developed. Light from the target diverges and is made parallel by the collimating lens.

Power drum

This is a drum marked from 0 to 20, plus and minus, which indicates the lens power when the lens is in focus. It physically moves the target up and down the focusing system.

Some power drums have no markings, merely being a focusing wheel. The power of the lens under test is displayed on a screen inside the instrument which is visible through the viewing telescope.

Cylinder axis wheel

The cylinder axis wheel controls the rotation of the target axis and indicates lens axis from 0° to 180°. It is not found in a ring-of-dots focimeter, although it is found in the hybrid models.

Frame table

The table holds spectacles in an exact 180° position. It is moved down, out of the way, for marking up uncut lenses.

Table control

This moves frame table up or down to locate the vertical lens centre.
Now that we have considered the main components of the focimeter, let's look at how the instrument works.

Table 8.1: Summary of focimeter parts

Parts	Functions
Observation system	
Eyepiece	The eyepiece can be focused to suit each user's vision.
Objective	The objective lens combines with the eyepiece to form an afocal system.
Graticule	Measures the power and direction of prism usually up to 5Δ. Also carries axis markings.
Prism cell	Holds auxiliary prisms to measure prisms over 5Δ.
Clamp	Holds the lens against the lens rest.
Marking device	Contains pins which dot the optical centre and horizontal meridian.
Focusing system	
Collimating lens	Makes divergent light from the target parallel.
Lens rest	Lens is held by the clamp against this aperture to measure its power.
Ink well	A container which supplies ink for the marking device (some focimeters have self-inking markers).
Power drum	A drum which moves the target. It may also carry the lens power measuring scale ($-20D$ to $+20D$).
Cylinder axis wheel	Controls the rotation of the target axis and indicates lens axis from $0°$ to $180°$ (not ring-of-dots focimeters)
Lens table	Holds spectacles in an exact $180°$ position.
Table control	Moves lens table up or down to locate vertical lens centre.
Power scale	Indicates lens power. If it is not shown on the power wheel it is located inside the instrument and viewed through the observation system.

Optical system of a focimeter

The focusing system is designed to produce an infinitely distant image. The lens in the focusing system of the instrument (see Figure 8.2) is called the collimating lens or 'standard lens', and has a power of+22.00 or +27.00 dioptres, depending on the manufacturer. This power simply has to be greater than the power of the highest plus lens which the instrument is designed to record, normally $+20D$ or $+25D$.

Within the focusing system there is a target, placed in front of the light source. The target appears as illuminated dots or crossed lines, depending on its design. Its movement is adjustable when you turn the power drum, and it can be rotated when you turn the axis adjustment. The target is geared to a scale where its movement, in terms of dioptres, is recorded.

When the focimeter is set at zero, or piano, light diverging from the target is made parallel by the standard lens. It then enters the viewing system, is brought to a focus at the graticule, diverges again and emerges at the other end as parallel light. At the lens where your eye is viewing, this light produces a bright, crisp image of the target at the other end of the instrument.

The viewing system is designed like a telescope and has an adjustable eyepiece.

You should never use a focimeter until you have adjusted the eyepiece for your eye, and have checked that the target is in focus with the power drum at zero.

The graticule, which is positioned at the second principal focal plane of the objective lens of the telescope, has a cross-line scale which can be rotated through 180°. The prism is often measured on concentric circles calibrated in prism dioptres. The crossed lines are geared to an internal protractor or an external drum from which the cylinder axis of an astigmatic lens may be read.

In recent years the telescope observation system has been replaced on some instruments by a projection system which projects an image of the target onto a screen. This permits the use of both eyes, reduces eye fatigue, and enables lens checking by two or more observers. Some models, as you will see later on, offer digital displays of the lens power and axis, while others offer a completely computerised operation in which a video monitor displays an automatic neutralisation of the lens, and supplies a print-out of the complete details of the lens powers.

Let us now consider what happens when a spectacle lens is placed at the lens rest. An unknown plus lens will converge light being transmitted from the focusing system before it enters the viewing system. A minus lens, of course, will diverge light before it enters the viewing system. Thus in both cases, a blurred target will appear. To measure the power of the unknown plus lens, you must turn the power drum to move the target closer to the standard lens. Light from the target will become increasingly too divergent for the standard lens to neutralise, or make parallel. Now the plus lens which lies between the standard lens and the viewing system will tend to converge the diverging light rays back to parallel. You will know this because the target will start to become clearer until it forms a bright, crisp focus. At this point you have a precise, clear power reading of the unknown plus lens. If, for example, the power drum reads +5.00, you know you have a spherical lens of +5.00 dioptres.

Of course, in the case of an unknown minus lens, the power barrel is turned to move the target away from the standard lens. Light from the target will not be divergent enough for the standard lens to make it parallel. The unknown minus lens, however, will tend to diverge the converging rays back to parallel, and the target will start to become clearer until it forms a bright, crisp focus.
Now that we have considered the focusing and viewing systems of a focimeter, we will now look at the target types.

Target types

There are two main types of focimeter target markings in general use, the 'ring-of-dots' (or corona) target, sometimes referred to as the European target, and the 'crossed-line' (or American) target. The recognition of each is clear by their names. Some focimeters use a hybrid of both corona and the cross-line.

Ring-of-dots target or 'corona' target

The ring-of-dots target takes the form of a ring of very small dots superimposed over a graticule target indicating a standard axis notation protractor reading from 0° to 180° anticlockwise.

When an astigmatic lens is under test and the target is in focus for either of the principal powers, each dot appears to be drawn out into a focal line which is at right angles to the meridian of power which creates them. When checking a spherical lens, the target remains a ring of dots.

A ring-of-dots focimeter has no need for an axis drum since the focal lines automatically line up along the axis or the power meridian, and the axis is measured by using the graticule.

Crossed-line target

As the name implies, this target has two sets of lines crossed at 90° to each other. In order to read the axis off the axis drum; it is necessary to understand which of the sets of lines that the manufacturer nominates to be the spherical reading. We will see, however, that you can check the power of the lens without knowing the correct lines to use for the 'sphere' power. The crossed-line target cannot form a sharp image of either set of straight lines until the lines are parallel to one of the principal meridians of the lens. The axis drum must be turned to make the lines unbroken.

A number of new models feature a 'ring-of-dots' target superimposed over a crossed-line target (a hybrid target). This focimeter is designed to appeal to the users who prefer the ring-of-dots and those who like the crossed-line target.

The three-step rule discussed below can be used to work out the lens power on any focimeter, regardless of its target type.

Types of focimeter

We have examined the telescopic type of focimeter, the most common type. There are, however, two other types of focimeter that deserve mention.

The projection focimeter allows the operator to view a screen from a distance (of about 0.5*m*). It enables the operator to use both eyes and is more comfortable for some users. The screen, however, can be difficult to see in a brightly lit room. The target and graticule, as they appear on the screen, are the same as the telescopic focimeter and the operation of the focimeter is the same. One word of caution, though, is that they often sit vertically and the frame table is often on the other side of the spectacles from the user. That is, the spectacles sit on the lens rest facing straight up with the top of the eye-wire nearest to the user.

The computerised focimeter is the most automated of all. The operator needs only to set the lenses or spectacles up on centre and to push a button. The focimeter will then read the power (and the prismatic effect and in some cases the PD) and print

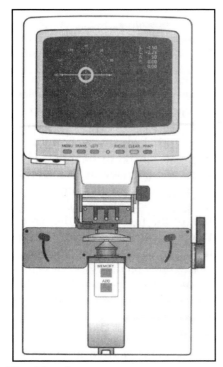

out the result. This type of focimeter is popular in hospital outpatient eye clinics and reception areas for ophthalmologists or with optometrists who can have their clerical staff neutralise a patient's spectacles before the consultation. Like the projection focimeter, caution should be taken when using the frame table; they have a similar set-up.

Both of these also make neutralising front seg multifocals difficult to measure, as the frame-temples cannot be opened out of the way. They obstruct the reading.

Figure 8.3: A typical digital
computerised focimeter

Checking lens power

The steps outlined below will work on any manual focimeter. Remembering the steps will mean that you do not need to search for the user's manual of the focimeter in order to check lenses on an unfamiliar focimeter. Before we look at the procedure for checking lenses, there are some general points that should be considered when using any telescopic focimeter.

1 First you should adjust the angle of the focimeter on the workbench, so the eyepiece is in a comfortable position.
2 Then check that the eyepiece is focused for your eye as we discussed earlier.
3 Finally, and this is the area some people have difficulty with, you should look into the eyepiece with both eyes open. This is to ensure that both eyes are parallel and that you are not converging and, therefore, accommodating.

To expand on that last point, you should use your dominant eye to look into the eyepiece. It is much easier to ignore the image in your non-dominant eye. To find your dominant eye simply focus on a distant object such as a door frame, with both eyes open. Hold your finger at arm's length and line it up with the distant object, as though it were the sight of a gun. Now close one eye. If the finger remains lined up with the object, you have closed your non-dominant eye; if the finger moves to the side, you have closed your dominant eye. That is, you have subconsciously selected your dominant eye to line up the finger with the object and have ignored the image of the non-dominant eye. If you carry out the exercise again and think about what you are seeing, you will be aware that you are seeing two images of your finger (if you only see one finger, you must see two objects because you are focused on your finger, not on the distant object — unless, of course, you are blind in one eye).

Checking spherical lenses

As you know, the fundamental characteristic of a spherical lens is to bring parallel rays of light to a single-point focus. When spherical lenses are placed on a focimeter we are simply measuring their capacity to converge light in the case of plus lenses, and diverge light in the case of minus lenses. The steps for measuring spherical lenses are:

1 Set up the vertometer for your own eyesight and comfortable viewing position.

2 Place the concave or back surface of the lens against the lens rest.

3 Raise the frame table if the lens is fitted into a frame, until it supports the frame.

4 Release the lens holder arm and support the lens securely against the lens stop.

5 Rotate the power drum towards the plus readings with the lens in position. If the target becomes clear and crisply focused, this is the power you need. If the target becomes more blurred, rotate the power drum back towards the minus readings until the target becomes clear and sharp. (In the ring-of-dots model, the dots will form a sharp 'corona' while in a crossed-line model, all the lines will be sharp.)

6 Note down the lens power on the drum. You have now checked a spherical lens.

Note: Always move the lens so that the target appears in the centre of the graticule if possible.

Checking cylindrical and sphero-cylindrical lenses

Few people have trouble checking spherical lenses on an unfamiliar focimeter but many, if not most balk at checking sphero-cylindrical lenses. But, it is not that hard and you don't need to reach for the manual. There is a simple three-step rule that works every time. Commit it to memory, it is the most important rule you could remember.

The three-step rule: crossed-line focimeter

Beware of unfamiliar focimeters they lie!

If you are using a crossed-line type focimeter that you are not used to then you will have a 50 per cent chance of being 90° off axis. Unless you know the lines that the manufacturer has determined for the sphere power, you cannot be sure that the axis drum is telling you the truth. If you use the three steps below you will always be correct, regardless of the focimeter you use. The three-step rule requires faith, though. Don't be tempted to look at the axis drum!

1 The first reading is your sphere power.

2 The second reading minus the first reading is your cyl. If you don't like doing the arithmetic, the direction you turn the power drum also indicates the sign of the cyl. If you turn towards minus you are measuring minus cyl—if you turn

towards plus you are measuring plus cyl.

3 The direction of lines at your second reading is your axis. Use the graticule to determine the direction of the lines. Once again, if you are using an unfamiliar crossed-line target, **don't** look at the axis drum. You will, though, need to rotate the axis drum to make the lines unbroken.

Corona focimeter (ring-of-dots)

If you are using a ring-of-dots focimeter, the first reading will simply be the point where the ring of dots first stretches into a clear set of lines.

It doesn't matter which reading is your first reading, but if you like to measure all of your powers with a minus cyl, simply select the stronger plus reading or the weakest minus reading as your 'first reading'.

If you are using a crossed-line or hybrid target you will, as I said, need to rotate the axis drum to make the lines unbroken, but **don't** look at the reading on the axis drum.

Once again, if you like to measure all of your powers with a minus cyl, simply select the stronger plus reading or the weakest minus reading as your 'first reading'.

Note: Always measure astigmatic lenses in the centre of the graticule with ring-of-dots focimeters. It may not always be possible to do this, especially with prism or progressive lenses, but try.

Let's consider some examples.

Fig.8.4: Example 1 - ring of dots
(a) (first reading)   **(b) second reading**

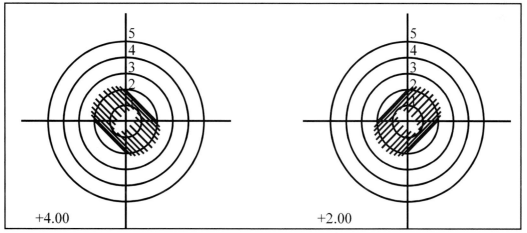

+4.00   +2.00

1 Your first reading is +4.00
2 Your second reading (+2.00) minus your first reading (+4.00) is your cyl.
   So +2.00 − +4.00 = −2.00 (here you are turning the power drum towards minus (+4.00 to +2.00), so you will get minus cyl.
3 The direction of the lines at the second reading is your axis (45°).
So the power is +4.00/−2.00 × 45.

Fig.8.5: Example 2 - crossed-line target

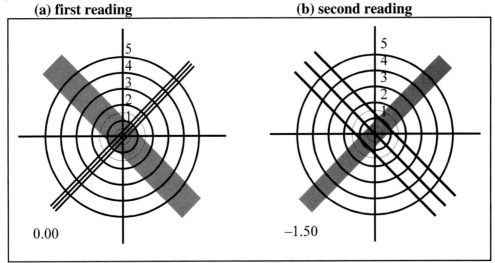

(a) first reading   (b) second reading

0.00   −1.50

1 Your first reading is plano.

2 Your second reading (−1.50) minus your first reading (0) is your cyl.
So −1.50 − −0 = −1.50 (here again you are turning the power drum towards minus (plano to −1.50), so you will get minus cyl.

3 The direction of the lines at the second reading is your axis (135°).
So the power is plano/−1.50 × 135.

If you were using a crossed-line target and, after using the three-step rule, you look at the axis drum and it tells you that the axis is 45 when the three-step rule has given you 135, you are right and the focimeter is wrong. It simply means that, for your first reading, you didn't use the lines the manufacturer designed for the sphere. If it makes you feel more comfortable, you can turn the axis drum through 90° and it will agree with you.

Checking a prism

The graticule is used to set up a lens for ordered prism or to determine the amount of prism in a completed pair of spectacles. It operates on the same principle as the tangent scale— that is, it measures the displacement of the target against a scale (the graticule). It also operates on the 'what you see is what you get' principle. Some people confuse themselves by remembering that you move a minus lens out to obtain base in prism as opposed to a plus lens which you move in. But, you don't need to consider this; if the target appears to be in, that is, towards the nasal, it is base in (if it were a minus lens you would have been pushing the lens out to get the target to move in). Simply imagine the spectacles looking at you and consider the position of the target.

Example

Figure 8.6 shows a crossed-line target with a spherical right lens for 2Δ base up and 3Δ base in as they would appear in a focimeter. The most important reference in positioning a prismatic lens is the central point where the lines intersect (or the centre of the ring of dots). The number on the graticule's circle shows the displacement in prism dioptres (Δ). The dotted lines shown extend vertically and horizontally from the target origin to coincide in the right lens with 2Δ base up and 3Δ base in, on the graticule. The target is displaced in the direction in which the base of the prism is desired.

Figure 8.6: Checking a prism

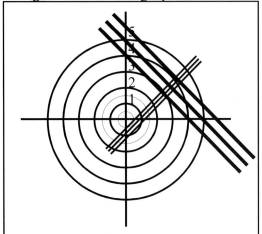

Checking the centres of finished spectacles

When you are checking a pair lenses fitted to a frame, the marked centre dots can be measured with PD ruler to test the accuracy of the lens centres according to the prescription, and the patient's measurements. If prism is ordered, the lenses should be dotted with the prescribed prism and the distance between the dots, which should be the PD, measured.

Dotting bifocal centres

The bifocal centres should not be dotted as we have dotted the distance centres. If you did dot the 'optical centre' of the near in this way, you would also have the effect of the distance power—that is, for a plus prescription the distance power would contribute base out prism to the seg and a minus lens would contribute base in prism. We are, however, interested in the optical centre of the seg (not the near, combined power). To find this we simply find the geometric centre of the seg.

This is a common error with trainee dispensing opticians. They dot the near centres using the focimeter and note that it does not correspond to the ordered near CD. It won't, of course, unless the distance section is piano.

Measuring multifocal additions

For multifocals with the seg on the front surface the following method should be used to measure the addition:

1 Measure the near front-vertex power (with the front surface of the lens against the lens rest).
2 Measure the distance front-vertex power (with the front surface of the lens against the lens rest).

The addition is the first reading minus the second.

To confirm the distance power you should measure the distance portion in the usual way (back-vertex power).

Figure 8.7: Measuring multifocal additions

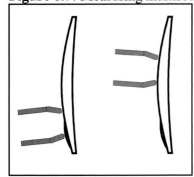

We measure the add this way because we want to determine the power of the seg, independent of the distance power. Its job is to make the divergent light from the near object parallel, so we need its power alone. If we measure the power at the back vertex, the seg is not against the lens rest and so effectivity gives an incorrect reading for the add. This is because we are actually measuring the effective power of the seg through the thickness of the distance lens.

Checking incorrectly, back-vertex, will generally give the correct result but, if the lens is reasonably thick (such as a high plus lens) the add will be incorrect. Many spectacles have been wrongly rejected and sent back to the laboratory because they were checked the wrong way.

If the seg is on the back, the addition is simply the difference between the back-vertex distance power and the back-vertex near power.

The procedure for checking trifocals is the same as that applying to bifocals. When measuring trifocal lenses with the trifocal formed on the front of the lens, follow exactly the same procedure suggested for measuring a bifocal. Make notes of the reading through the reading segment, through the intermediate band, and through the distance, all front-vertex. Almost all trifocals are designed so that the intermediate power is half the power of the reading addition.

In the past, some observers have noted that if we were to make up readers from a prescription such as +3.00*D* distance with a +2.50*D* add, we would make up lenses with a power of +5.50*D*. That is, the lenses would have a back vertex power of +5.50*D*. Yet, if the lenses were made up as bifocals or progressives we are not interested in the back-vertex power through the seg and, indeed, it wouldn't be +5.50*D*. Why is this so? Is the bifocal checking method wrong? The official answer is that both are correct. Let's look at the reasoning.

As mentioned above, bifocals are checked the way they are because we want to see the effect of the seg alone. If the seg is not against the lens rest, effectivity will come into play if we compare the two back-vertex measurements (distance and near). The theory is that the add (or the seg) is meant to render parallel the divergent light from the near object. If, when testing the eyes, the refractionist had the distance power in the trial frame and then added a plus lens (the add) to the front cell of the trial frame (using our example, a +2.50 is placed in front of the +3.00), the bifocal checking method is closest to what the refractionist has done since the seg on the front surface is essentially doing the same thing. The way we make single-vision readers would then, theoretically, be wrong. On the other hand, if the refractionist set up the reading power as a single lens, using our example (a +5.50 lens is placed in the trial frame or refractor head), one could argue that the back vertex of the reading power is +5.50 and so the bifocal seg should read this power back-vertex. Thus, our single-vision readers would have the correct power.

9. OPHTHALMIC PRISMS

Prisms are usually incorporated in a spectacle correction when the patient has some kind of muscle imbalance known as a phoria. This simply means that the patient cannot fuse the two separate images from the individual eyes without some kind of help. By apparently displacing the image from one or both eyes, a prism enables the images to overlap.

Prisms can be incorporated into a spectacle prescription as a separately stated components or they can be produced by an appropriate decentration of the lens. This is dealt with later. It can be seen that unwanted prismatic effects can be induced by the incorrect centring of lenses. It is important therefore that lenses are centred correctly for the appropriate task in order to avoid undesirable prismatic effects and consequently symptoms of strain or double-vision.

One very important point to remember with ophthalmic prisms is that they have both *magnitude* and *direction.* It is meaningless to state one without the other.

> e.g.   R. +3.00*DS*/+0.75*DC* × 180 2 Δ base UP
> L. +2.50*DS*/+0.50*DC* × 175 2 Δ base DOWN.

A *plano prism* is nothing more than a wedge-shaped piece of transparent material. Both surfaces are plane and therefore there is no focal power. If we produce a plano prism as a lens, then the two surfaces have the same radii of curvature, as in a plano sphere, but are inclined at an angle to one another [Fig.9.1]. The edge **AA´** is known as the *refracting edge* or *apex,* with angle α being the *apical angle.* The thick edge is known as the *base.*

Fig.9.1   **[a] a plano prism**   **[b] a principal section**   **[c] a meniscus plano prism**

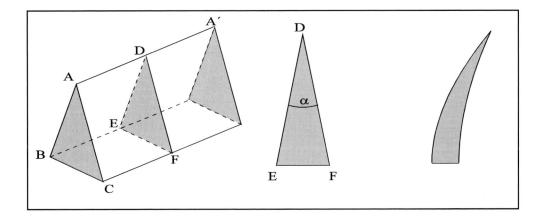

The essential property of a plano prism is that it *deviates*, or changes the direction of, light rays passing through it. An object viewed through a plano prism is therefore seen in a different direction from that in which it would appear if viewed without the prism. If you view a cross line chart and apply the rotation test as described in the previous chapter, the crossline will appear to be displaced towards the apex of the prism as shown in Fig.9.2[a]. When the prism is rotated the crosslines appear to rotate with it Fig.9.2[b] & [c]. If the transverse test is applied, no movement is observed. It should be noted that the greater the distance of the crossline chart from the prism, the greater the displacement, but we will cover the reasons for this a little later.

Fig.9.2 A crossline chart when viewed through a rotated prism

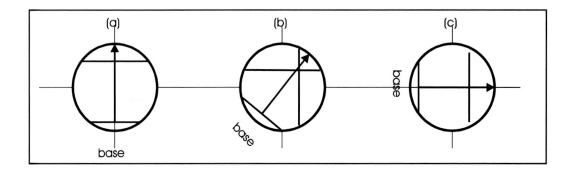

Units

.

There are many units of angle. The one which is most well known and used is the degree based on the division of a circle into 360 equal sectors.

For mathematical and scientific use, such as with computers, a different system of angular measurement is employed. With this system, which is known as *circular measure*, an angle is defined in terms of a pure number, the ratio of two lengths. In Fig.9.3, **OA** is a line pivoted at **O**. If it is rotated about **O** to the new position **OA´**, the angle θ through which it has turned would be expressed in circular measure as the ratio of the length of arc **AA´** to the radius **OA.** The unit of angle, termed a *radian*, is therefore that angle in which the length of arc is equal to the radius [i.e. AA' = OA].

If we consider a complete circle, the length of arc is a complete circumference, which is equal to 2π times the radius. Therefore:

$$2\pi \text{ rad} = 360\,°, \text{ making } 1 \text{ rad} = 180/\pi \text{ degrees}$$
and $1 \text{ degree} = \pi/180 \approx 0.01745 \text{ rad.}$

Fig.9.3 Basis of 'circular measure'

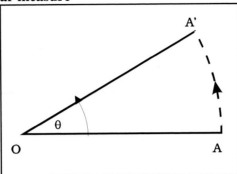

For ophthalmic optics, yet another unit, the *prism dioptre* [Δ] has been devised. The prism dioptre is a unit of angular measure, being the angle whose tangent is 1/100. A prism of power 1 Δ produces a displacement of 1 unit on a scale placed at 100 units from the prism. An angle θ can be expressed in prism dioptres simply by multiplying its tangent by 100. E.g. if θ is 10 degrees, then

$$\theta \text{ in } \Delta = 100 \text{ x tan } 10\,^{\circ} = 100 \text{ x } 0.17633 = 17.63 \text{ } \Delta$$

The deviation *d* undergone by a ray passing through a plano prism of apical angle *a* is affected by:

1. the angle of incidence
2. the apical angle of the prism
3. the refractive index **n** of the material, which as we mentioned in an earlier chapter, varies with the wavelength of the light under consideration.

Ophthalmic prisms rarely exceed an apical angle of 10°. The power of an ophthalmic prism is defined as the deviation it produces, expressed in prism dioptres, on a ray incident normally on one surface, the wavelength specified [587 *nm*] corresponding to the d-line of the helium spectrum.

When we consider prisms of low power, the relationship between deviation and apical angle is given to a sufficient degree of accuracy by the approximate formula:

$d=[n - 1]a$ which can also be written as

$$\tan a = \frac{\tan d}{(n-1)} = \frac{P}{100(n-1)} \text{ where } P \text{ is the power of the prism.}$$

Unfortunately, this is not quite accurate enough in all cases. The exact relationship between the apical angle *a* of a prism and the deviation *d* when the incidence is normal is:

$$\tan a = \frac{\sin d}{n - \cos d} \text{ which can be put in the following more}$$

convenient form:

$$\tan a = \frac{P}{100(n-1)+nP^2/200}$$

Fig.9.4 Deviation [*d*] and apparent displacement [*y*] produced by a plano prism.

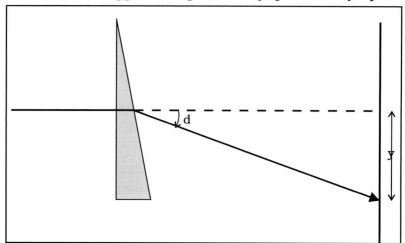

Prism thickness difference

Fig.9.5 shows a principal section through a flat plano prism. The difference between the edge thickness *p* at the apex of the prism and the edge thickness *q* at the base of the prism is termed the *prism thickness difference*. In the diagram it is denoted by *g*.

Fig.9.5 Prism thickness difference

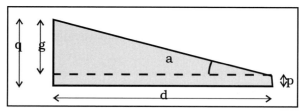

For a given apical angle there is clearly a relationship between the prism thickness difference and the diameter over which it is measured. Hence, when grinding a prism the apical angle can be controlled by working to a pre-determined thickness difference over a specified diameter. From the definition of a prism dioptre:

$$a\Delta = \frac{100g}{d}$$

hence $\qquad P = \frac{100g(n-1)}{d} \qquad$ and $\qquad g = \frac{Pd}{100(n-1)}$

Prism base setting

The object of an ophthalmic prism is to produce a displacement, in a specified direction, of the images seen through it. As previously stated, the direction of image displacement is always towards the apex of the prism. Hence to produce a displacement upwards, any base-apex line must be vertical, with the base of the prism below the apex, i.e. down. It has become an accepted standard in practice to use the base of a prism to specify its setting in relation to the eye. This is known as the **base** *setting* and can be defined as the direction from apex to base. The current method of specifying a base setting is either by denoting *up* or *down* if in the vertical direction, or by *in* or *out* if in the horizontal direction. *In* is always taken as being towards the nose with both eyes. If an oblique base setting is to be specified then the 360° notation as illustrated in Fig.9.6 is used.

Fig.9.6 The 360° protractor

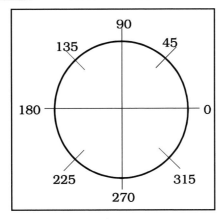

It can be seen that using this system *up* relates to 90° and *down* to 270°, whereas for the right eye *in* and *out* are 0° and 180° respectively. For the left eye *in* and *out* relate to 180° and 0° respectively.

Dividing or splitting prisms

If a prescription specifies a prism in one eye only, the same effect can be obtained by dividing the prism between the two eyes as its purpose is to correct a binocular condition - uncompensated heterophoria. This can be useful to balance and reduce thickness and weight where the prescriptions are similar in the two eyes. Where one lens is much stronger in one eye than the other, it may be better to balance thickness and weight by introducing all or most of the prism into the weaker lens. On the other hand it may be easier and cheaper to produce the prism in the stronger lens merely by decentration.

That part of the original prism which is transferred to the other eye must always have its base direction reversed, bearing in mind that base out for one eye is opposite in direction to base out for the other eye, and similarly with base in. For example : R.E. 4 Δ base out would become, when equally divided:

	R.E. 2 Δ base out	L.E. 2 Δ base out
or	R.E. 2 Δ base 180	L.E. 2 Δ base 0

on the other hand L.E. 4 Δ base up would become:

	R.E. 2 Δ base down	L.E. 2 Δ base up
or	R.E. 2 Δ base 270	L.E. 2 Δ base 90

59

Compounding and resolving prisms

Prescriptions occasionally call for a vertical prism in conjunction with a horizontal one, the net result or *resultant prism* will of course be at some oblique angle. Let us consider the prescription L.E. 3 Δ base down with 4 Δ base out.

To find the resultant prism, draw **OV** vertically 3 units in length and **OH** horizontally 4 units in length on the same scale [Fig.9.7] Complete the rectangle. The diagonal **OR** then represents both the magnitude and direction of the resultant prism which is found to be L.E. 5 Δ base 323 It could be measured from an accurately drawn construction, or calculated as follows.

Fig.9.7 Graphical construction for compounding prisms

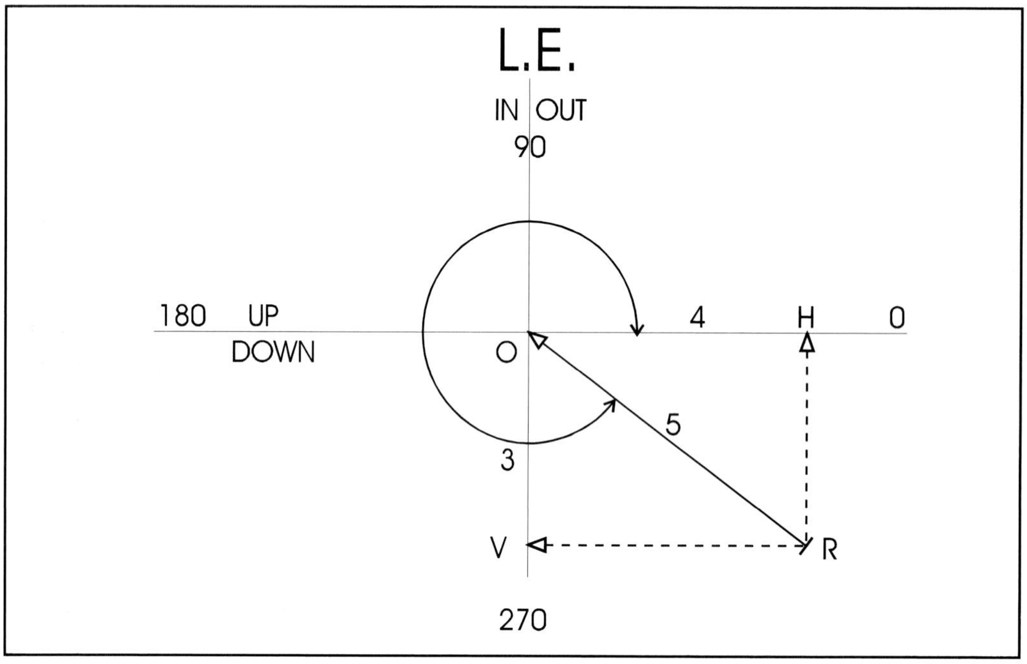

Using Pythagoras' theorem, from the triangle **OVR**

$$OR^2 = OV^2 + VR^2 \quad \therefore OR^2 = 3^2 + 4^2 = 25 \quad \therefore OR = \sqrt{25} = 5$$

$$\tan V\hat{R}O = OV \div VR \ = 3 \div 4 = 0.75 \quad \therefore V\hat{R}O = 37° \text{ or } 323°$$

The process of finding the single resultant prism which replaces two given prisms with different base settings is known as *compounding* prisms. The reverse process whereby the vertical and horizontal components of a single oblique prism are found is called *resolving*.

10. FACIAL MEASUREMENTS

Before ordering prescription glasses, or indeed even before carrying out a visual examination, the distance between the pupils must be determined. This distance is known as the *interpupillary distance*, or P.D. It can be measured in a variety of ways.

However, firstly, let us look at the visual axes.

Visual axes

Visual axes are imaginary lines, which pass through the nodal point and macula of the eye. The macula is the part of the light-sensitive retina where we see things most distinctly and lies at the posterior pole of the eye. The nodal point is one of the cardinal points of an optical system, and is the point in the eye through which all light rays pass on their way to form an image on the retina. When you look at something, you point your visual axis at it, and in this way the image of what you are looking at falls on the macula and is seen in greatest detail. You may think of the visual axes as the 'lines of sight'. Objects off to the side of what you look at form images which are not seen in as great detail, and in fact are very blurry.

The visual axes lie slightly to the nasal side of the optical axes (see Figure 10.1). That is, the visual axis does not pass through the centre of the pupil but, rather, through a point a little to the nasal side. This is why the reflection seen in a pupillometer does not appear to be in the pupil centre and why the pupillometer's PD is slightly smaller than the PD taken by a PD rule. It is the pupillometer's measurement that we want. It is measuring the distance between the visual axes.

Fig.10.1

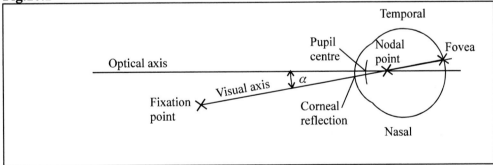

Interpupillary distance

In this section we will focus on measuring interpupillary distance and the techniques used to do this. Interpupillary distance, or pupillary distance (PD) as it is commonly known, is usually defined as the distance between a patient's pupil centres, when the patient is effectively looking at a distant object. More correctly, it is the distance between the visual axes.

Accurate PD measuring is necessary for placing the optical centres of the lenses directly in front of our patient's pupil (at least horizontally) to avoid unprescribed prism. Let's now examine the methods and their advantages and disadvantages.

Using the pupillometer

The pupillometer is the only instrument designed to measure the distance between the visual axes and not merely the pupil centres.

The term pupillometer is something of a misnomer since a pupillometer, technically, is an instrument that measures the area of a pupil. Nevertheless the term is more commonly used for the instrument that measures the PD. It is also known as a corneal reflex pupillometer.

The pupillometer uses a corneal reflex and is equipped with a battery powered light source. The patient looks at a green circle (usually) within the machine, and fixates at preset distances from $35cm$ to infinity. This instrument is best used by asking your patient to hold it as though it were a pair of binoculars and look through the eyepieces in the end with the nose pads. The nose pads balance the pupillometer in a similar fashion to a spectacle frame, and allow you to place your thumbs on the pads which move the thin wires you see in the instrument when you look through your single eyepiece.

The internal light produces a reflection on each cornea. Move the thin wires until you see them bisect the bright corneal reflection. You can perform this task on your patient's eyes individually because the instrument has an occluding device.

These monocular measurements are accepted as the client's line of sight, but are really an objective measurement of the position of corneal reflection. The reflection of the light source from the anterior surface of the cornea, which is used to measure the PD, is slightly toward the nasal, resulting in a measurement approximately $1mm$ smaller than a PD rule measurement. The visual axis is usually displaced by about 5° towards the nasal; thus the pupil centre is not accurate. The following are the steps to take when using a pupillometer to measure monocular PDs.

1. Set the instrument for distance or near readings. It is important that the setting be checked before use. It is not uncommon to find that the previous user has left the instrument on a near setting, having completed the near centration measurement last.

2. Ask your patient to hold the instrument as if looking through binoculars, and to look at the green circles.

3. Adjust the thumb pads until the thin wires are superimposed on the corneal reflex. The black line should pass through the very centre of the reflex.

4. Remove the instrument and read the right-eye and left-eye monocular PDs from the graduated scale. The binocular PD is also visible.

Binocular or monocular measurement

The pupillometer can measure the patient's PD with both eyes viewing the target or one eye at a time, occluding each eye in turn. The PD should be measured monocularly if the patient has strabismus.

Measuring the Interpupillary Distance

The anatomical interpupillary distance is the distance from the centre of one pupil to the centre of the other pupil, measured in millimetres [Fig.10.2].

Fig.10.2

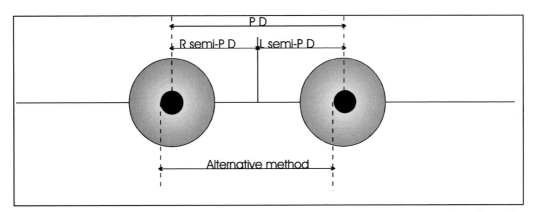

The purpose of determining the P.D. is so that we may accurately place the optical centres of the prescription lenses in front of the patient's eyes. Failure to do this will induce unwanted prismatic effects, requiring the wearer to turn his eyes inwards or even outwards, to keep from experiencing double vision. Over a long period of time, this error causes visual discomfort and can result in a decreased ability of the eyes to work together in binocular vision. When the wearer looks straight ahead, the visual axis of each eye should pass through or above the optical centre of each lens (more about heights will be discussed later).

The most common method used to measure the P.D. involves the least amount of equipment, The technique uses a simple millimetre rule, commonly referred to as a P.D. rule.

The dispensing optician positions himself directly in front of the subject whose P.D. is to be measured, at the same level and at a distance of about 50 *cm* [20 *ins*]. If the dispensing optician with a 70 *mm* P.D. is measuring a subject with a 50 *mm* P.D. then the maximum error will be about 1 *mm*. If the optician comes closer, say to about 25 *cm* then the error will double.

The P.D. rule is positioned across the subject's nose and resting against the spectacle frame which is to be used. We are then measuring the P.D. [strictly speaking this is the centration distance, which in most cases will be the same as the distance binocular P.D.] in the plane of the lenses. The dispensing optician holds the P.D. rule between thumb and forefinger, and steadies his hand by placing his remaining three fingers against the subject's head or using the longest to grip the back of the spectacle front.

The dispensing optician closes his right eye. The subject is instructed to look at the dispensing optician's open eye [or preferably a pen torch held *centrally* in front of it] while the dispensing optician lines up the zero mark with the centre of the subject's right corneal reflex. When the zero mark is lined up correctly, the dispensing optician closes his left eye and opens his right, again instructing the subject to look at his open eye [or pen torch]. The binocular P.D. for distance is read off at the mark falling in the centre of the subject's left corneal reflex.

When difficulty is experienced in determining the exact centre of the pupil, the edge of the pupil may be used as a measuring point if both pupils are the same size. Measurement is read from the *left side* of one pupil to the *left side* of the other pupil.

When a subject has dark irises or unequally sized pupils it may be difficult to use either centre or edge of the pupil. In such cases, the dispensing optician may use the limbus edge - the sharp demarcation between dark iris and white sclera. Again some caution is required as many subjects have about ½ *mm* of nasal eccentricity of the limbus, thus twice this amount needs to be deducted from the result obtained by this method.

Occasionally the person doing the measuring is unable to close one eye independently of the other. This can be remedied by covering the eye with the free hand. The practice of holding the lid down with one finger gives an unprofessional appearance, especially when wearing glasses! Occluding the eye with the hand held flat appears to be a natural part of the test and doesn't reveal a person's inability to close one eye only.

There are also various measuring gauges (other than the pupillometer) available which overcome the need for the operator to close one eye. They are of course more expensive than the P.D. rule and not so easily carried around.

Fig.10.3 Measurement of Distance Binocular P.D.

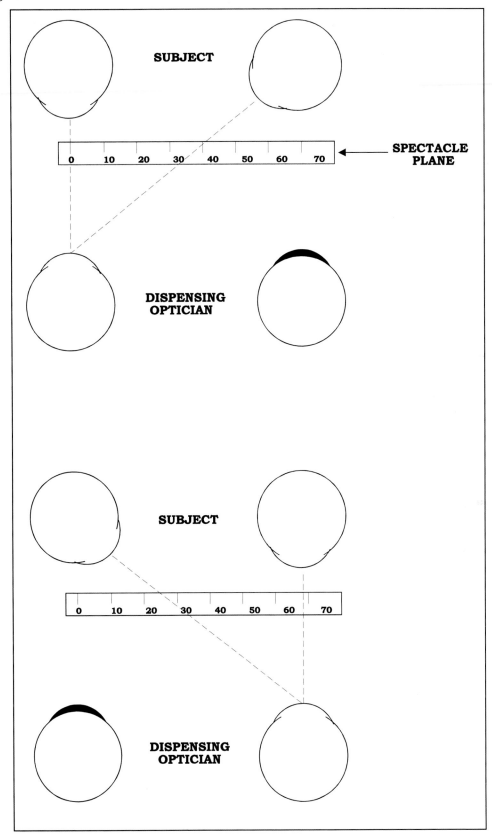

Since faces are not always symmetrical, it is often necessary to specify the interpupillary distance for each eye independently. The need for measurement of the monocular P.D. also arises in the fitting of multifocal lenses particularly progressive addition lenses. The monocular P.D. is taken by measuring from the centre of the bridge to the centres of the respective pupils. The procedure consists of the following three steps.

1. Measure the binocular P.D. as described above using the centre of the pupil as the reference point.

2. Before moving the rule, note the scale reading at the centre of the bridge. This is the right monocular P.D.

3. Subtract this reading from the binocular reading to obtain the left monocular P.D.

If the subject has an asymmetrical nose - such as when it has been broken - then the frame will position itself somewhat to the left or right. This is another good reason to measure PDs with the actual frame that will be worn

Measuring the Near Centration Distance

As we are interested in where to place the optical centres of the lenses it is vital that we measure the distance between the pupil centres in the plane of the lenses whilst the subject is fixating upon the object.

In order to achieve this the dispensing optician places himself at the subject's working or reading distance, and with his dominant eye as centrally as possible in line with the subject's nose. As before the dispensing optician closes his other eye and instructs the subject to look into his open eye. The centre of the subject's right pupil is lined up with the zero of the P.D. rule, which is of course being steadied against the frame to be worn. The centre of the subject's left pupil is then read off on the scale of the rule. Neither dispensing optician or subject are required to shift their gaze during this process. The result is the *near centration distance* as opposed to the near P.D. [see Fig.10.4]

Measuring heights

While most people consider heights an essential part of dispensing bifocals, progressives etc, they do not necessarily associate the measurement of heights with single-vision lenses—with the exception, perhaps, of dropping centres for readers. But, single-vision lenses also need to be set at a certain height—and not just aspherics. The manufacturers of aspheric lenses have made it clear that heights are an important part of fitting their lenses but the principle applies to any single-vision lens. The fact that many of us have not considered the measurement of heights for single-vision spherical and toroidal lenses is an indication of how forgiving those lenses were (or how tolerant their wearers were). It is true that it is more critical for aspheric lenses but, as you will see, the principle applies to any lens.

The principal axis/centre of rotation rule

The optical centre of a single-vision lens (not just aspherics) should be set so that the principal axis of the lens passes through the centre of rotation of the eye. This ensures the minimisation of the effects of aberrations such as marginal astigmatism. In order to do this the optical centre must be dropped below the pupil centre 1*mm* for every 2° of panto-scopic tilt. There are two ways we can take this measurement.

Method 1

1 Adjust the frame so that it is in its final fitting.
2 Measure the pantoscopic tilt. The easiest way to do this is to use the back of your wooden PD rule. The thin wobbly PD rules that are given away by lens and frame companies do not generally have this feature.
3 Place the frame on the client. With your head at the same level as your client's, determine the position of the centre of the pupil. This can be done with any of the three methods used for determining the bifocal or progressive heights, discussed in the next section.
4 Lower the height of the optical centre 1*mm* for every 2° of pantoscopic tilt.

The problem with this method is that it does not take into consideration the positioning of the wearer's ears.

Method 2

1 Adjust the frame
2 Have your client tilt their head back until the lenses are at 90° to the floor (see Figure 10.4).
3 While your client is holding their head in this position determine the centre of the pupil (using any of the three methods). This will produce the same result as method 2. When the client returns to a normal posture the optical centre position that you have marked will drop to the same position that you would have marked using method 1.

The advantages of the second method are that you do not have to be concerned that the person is sitting in a 'natural' position. It is very difficult to sit in a natural position when told to do so. Also, there is no chance of making an error when measuring the pantoscopic tilt.

While this must be done for aspheric lenses, it should, theoretically, be done for all single-vision distance spectacles to produce the ideal visual result. For lower-powered spherical and sphero-cyl lenses, however, the difference is not very significant and the cosmetic appearance of the completed spectacles may be better if the lenses are made up on the horizontal centre line.

Fig.10. 4 Locating the height for the optical centre

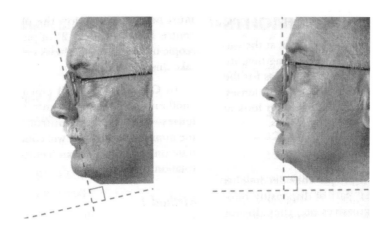

Fig.10.5 The relationship between vertical positioning of the optical centre and the pantoscopic angle.

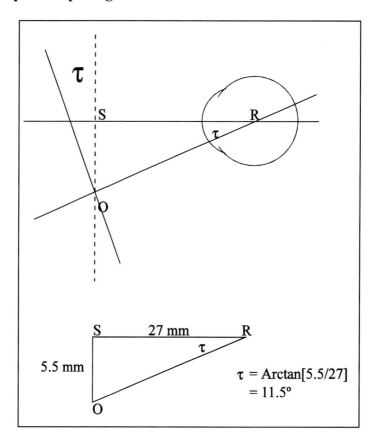

For each millimetre decentration down from the primary line of gaze the pantoscopic angle should be increased by about 2°.

Fig.10.6 Measurement of Near Centration Distance

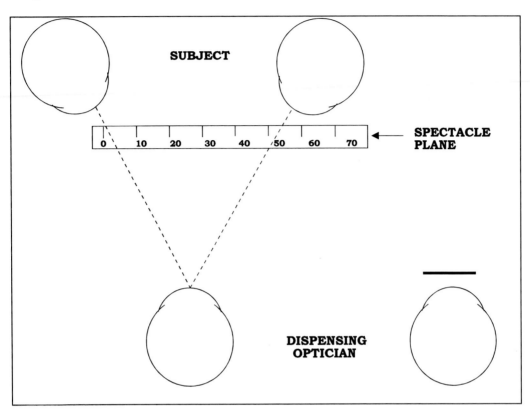

Fig.10.7 P.D. - Centration Distance Relationship

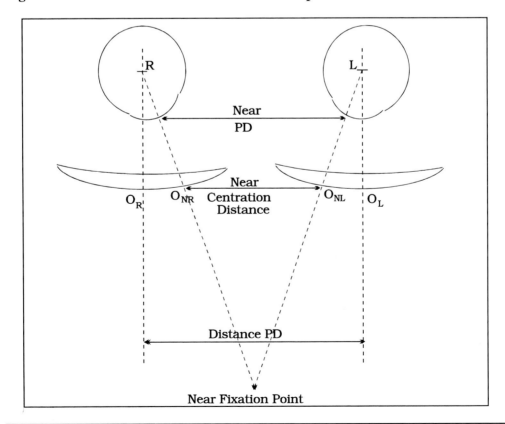

Facial Measurements

Facial measurements can be taken using the 'Fairbanks' facial measurement gauge. This gauge can be used for all the commonly taken facial measurements. It consists of a plastic ruler which has a rotating metal pointer fixed to it, and a cursor. [Fig.10.8].

Fig.10.8 The Fairbanks Facial Measurement Gauge

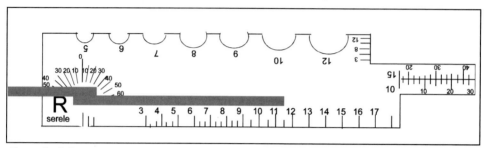

Crest height

This is the distance from the lower edge of the subject's iris to the bearing surface of the nose in the plane of the front.

Remove the cursor from the rule. Hold the narrow end of the rule horizontally on the estimated bearing surface of the nose [Fig.10.9]. Read off the crest height on the vertical scale against the lower edge of the subject's iris. Be sure to angle the rule slightly so that it sits in the same position as a spectacle frame. Right and left measurements can be taken which, if different, indicate that the two eyes are at different heights. The crest height is, however, recorded as a single measurement.

Bridge projection

This is the distance between the bearing surface of the nose and the tips of the eyelashes.

Place the cursor on the rule such that the cut-out edge is at the end of the rule and so that the transparent scale is over the section marked '+ -' on the rule. With the subject bending slightly forward, place the thin end of the rule against the estimated bearing surface and move the cursor until it just clears the lashes. Read off the position of the scale marks on the cursor against the scale on the rule. It is important to record the measurement as a '+' [projection] or a '-' [inset] as the case may be [Fig.10.10].

Apical radius

Place the front surface of the rule with cut out radii on the nose bearing surface and angled as before to simulate a spectacle frame front. Select the radius that fits best the bearing surface of the nose. If in doubt select the larger radius [Fig.10.11].

Fig.10.9 Crest height

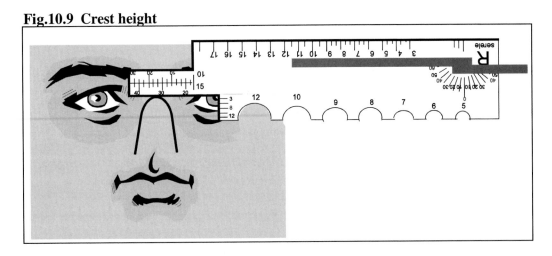

Fig.10.10 Bridge projection

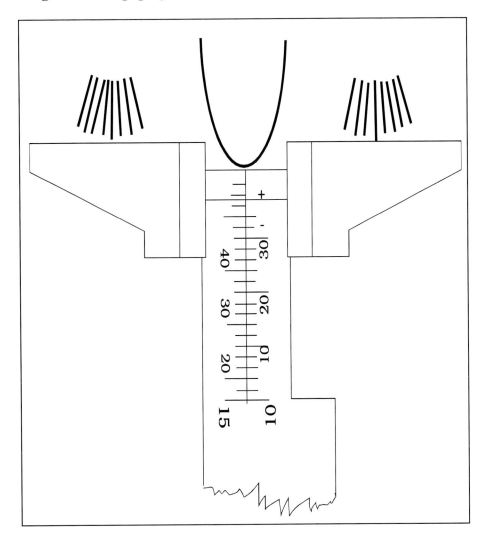

Fig.10.11 Apical radius

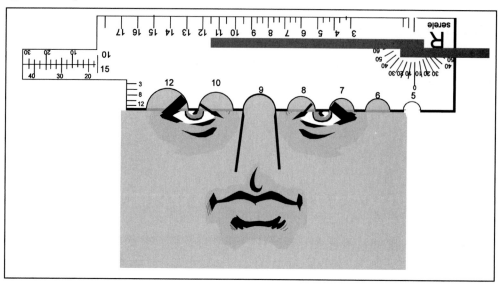

DBR @ 10 *mm* below crest

This the distance between the rims measured at a point 10 *mm* below the crest.

Hold the rule with the serrated edge uppermost and place the cursor on the thin end so that the cut-out edge of the cursor is facing outwards. Place the rule on the estimated bearing surface of the nose. Close the cursor so that it is just touching the nose on one side with the ruler touching the other side of the nose. The DBR at 10 is measured off on the scale marked '10'. Do not trap the nose too tightly and be sure to angle the rule[Fig.10.12].

Fig.10.12 DBR @ 10 *mm* below crest

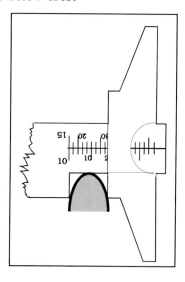

DBR @ 15 *mm* below crest

Repeat the above procedure but with the rule the other way up, taking the reading from the scale marked '15'[Fig.10.13].

Fig.10.13 DBR @ 15 *mm* below crest.

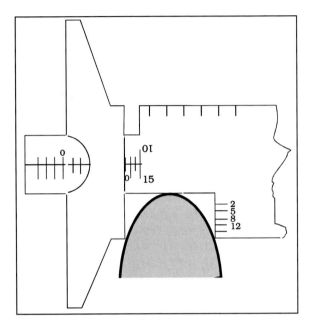

DBR on horizontal centre line

This is the width of the nose in the plane of the spectacle front in a line with the lower edge of the subject's iris.

Either of the above procedures can be used except that this time the lower edge of the rule is held in line with the lower edge of the iris. Readings can be taken on the '10' or '15' scale, whichever is best for the subject's shape of nose.

Frontal angle

Hold the rule on the nose in the plane of the front with the serrated edge uppermost, and the short end of the metal pointer projecting downwards. Rotate the short pointer until it rests against the estimated bearing surface of the bridge. Read off the frontal angle against the protractor scale [Fig.10.14].

Fig.10.14 Frontal angle

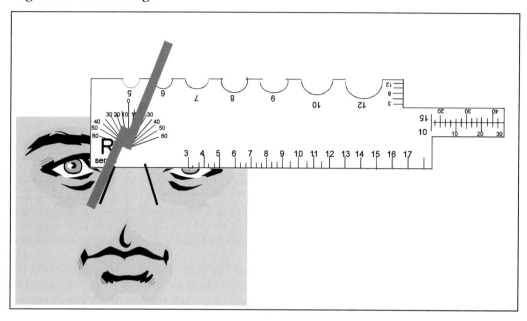

Splay angle

With the rule held horizontally and with its flat surface parallel to the floor, place the rule against the face so that the short end of the pointer is projecting straight towards the subject. With the subject bending his head forward, measure the angle at the estimated bearing surface. The rule should be approximately on a line through the lower edge of the subject's iris, which is taken as the horizontal centre line [Fig.10.15].

Fig.10.15 Splay angle

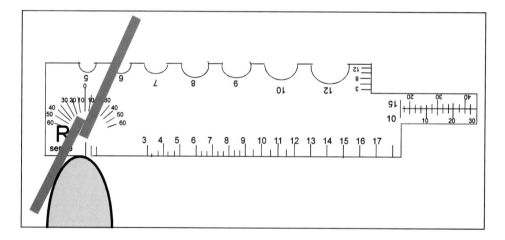

Length to bend

Hold the rule with the serrated edge uppermost, and the long end of the pointer projecting downwards at the same angle as the spectacle front will be, and at the same require distance from the lashes. The length to bend is read off on the rule at the top of the ear [Fig.10.16].

Fig.10.16 Length to bend

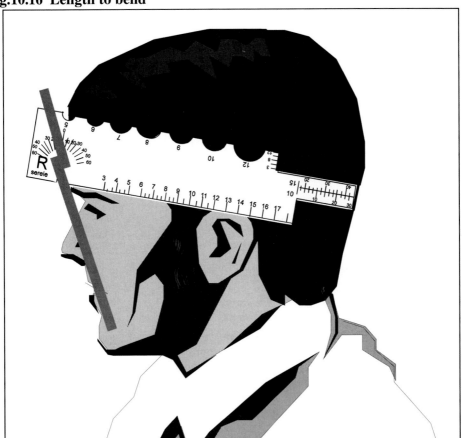

Head width

This is the measurement of the head at its widest point, usually at the ear point.

Two rules are required for this measurement. Hold the facial gauge with the serrated edge uppermost and the opposite edge resting lightly on the skull. The long arm of the metal pointer should project vertically downwards. Place the pointer in front of and just touching the right ear of the subject. The second rule or straight edge rests vertically on the opposite side of the head and where it crosses the scale of the facial gauge is the head width [Fig.10.17].

Fig.10.17 Head width

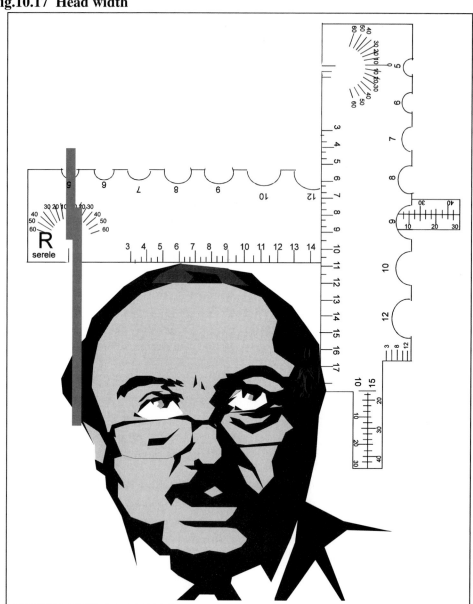

11. PAEDIATRIC DISPENSING

There is no clear understanding as to what is meant by paediatric dispensing: it is not an official term. It is clearly accepted, though, that a different approach needs to be taken when dealing with children. For the purposes of this chapter we will concentrate though on the age group 4 to 11.

What makes paediatric dispensing different? Why should it warrant a whole chapter to itself? Well, there are a number of answers to these questions.

1 There is what I like to call the 'duality of the patient'. That is, we are dealing with two patients, often with conflicting interests: the parent and the child. This duality requires some special skills from dispensing opticians that are not needed with an adult patient. Those of you with young children or siblings would have been aware of this 'conflict' any time you have visited the shoe shop or clothing store, hoping to select a pair of smart casual shoes only to see the child point to the 'outrageous' purple and black-striped boots.

2 Children tend to be rougher with themselves, their clothes and their spectacles than adults. We understand our frailty and, generally, treat ourselves with some care. Children, on the other hand, tend to act as if they were invincible. Indeed, they are more durable than us, increasing the gap between their durability and that of their clothes and spectacles.

3 Children are not merely small adults. Their facial features are quite different from a mature adult, requiring special frames. Dispensing opticians need to understand these differences and know how to fit a child correctly. Lens selection, too, involves special consideration, as does the taking of facial measurements.

4 Paediatric dispensing is fun. We are dealing with children; relax and enjoy. Of course, not all children will be happy and agreeable, as any primary school teacher will tell you. But, you are not dealing with a class of them. Some may not be happy with the thought of wearing glasses. In these cases the challenge is greater, but anyone who specialises in dispensing to children will tell you that the ups well outnumber the downs.

Until about the 1980s children were rarely given much thought when it came to dispensing spectacles or designing frames. Even if we discount altruistic motives, manufacturers and dispensing opticians had not recognised the market potential of children. Opticians had little to offer: frames were black or brown (or pink); two-tone or full-colour. The lenses were toughened glass—little glass bricks!

Spectacles were largely considered as medical appliances (for children). Indeed, even adults considered spectacles as a crutch for their vision. Adult spectacles, though, moved into the fashion field well before children's spectacles. Children were treated as miniature adults.

But, now we have designer frames and lightweight lenses for children. More children are wearing spectacles than before. We are testing children earlier and there is more screening being carried out. The link between learning difficulties and poor vision has been recognised. Children are less likely to have to struggle through school, unable to read comfortably or see the board.

THE CHANGING IMAGE OF SPECTACLES

Spectacles have been seen as a fashion accessory for adults for some time now and, increasingly, children are accepting them more positively. Many of their heroes wear spectacles. Films and television are now beginning to portray spectacles in a better light. No longer are they confined to the bookworm, the absent-minded professor, the nerd etc. We are now seeing models, sports people and the like wearing them.

But, while children view spectacles more positively, they are no longer content to wear what their parents tell them (if they ever were). Children today are more demanding and brand-conscious. We rarely see children wearing ordinary sandles or an unmarked cap.

Age differences

Children's' attitudes to spectacles vary with age. Younger children (up to about 8 or 9) are less likely to want spectacles than older children. Brightly coloured frames and spectacle cases, though, will often appeal to this age group. On the other hand, teens are more likely to recognise spectacles as an accessory and identify with adult spectacle wearers, such as models, musicians or actors.

Children up to the age of about 9 will generally consider themselves as children but, when is a child not a child? The answer is when he or she says so! You may have noticed, for example, that children of between around 9 and 12 will reject a children's menu when presented to them at a restaurant, and any crayons or puzzles handed to them is nothing short of an insult. If they do not like being treated as kids, then don't. They will not appreciate being taken to the kiddies' corner to select a frame so make sure that not all children's frames are in this area. Have some small sizes on your adult display.

FRAME SELECTION
Technical criteria

As I mentioned earlier, children are not merely scaled-down adults. Their facial features are shaped differently and they are constantly growing. In particular, young children do not have a developed nose. This is the most significant difference between the adult face and the child face. Manufacturers of good children's frames are aware of these differences and have incorporated the following characteristics in their designs.

Characteristics of good kids' frames
Lower crest

Because the child's nose is flatter and the bridge not properly developed, the crest of the bridge needs to be lower in children's frames. A scaled-down adult frame would cause the visual axis to pass through the very top of the lens.

Larger splay

Once again, the flat shape and lack of projection requires a larger splay.

Flatter pantoscopic tilt

The lack of projection from the face and the relative projection of the cheeks necessitates a flatter pantoscopic tilt. Too much tilt would cause the bottom rim to rest against the cheek.

Fig. 11.1 Larger splay   **Fig.11.2 Flatter pantoscopic tilt**

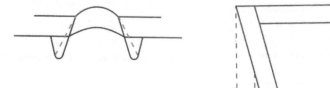

Fig.11.3 Lower crest

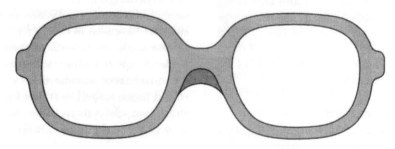

Fig.11.4 Larger frontal angle

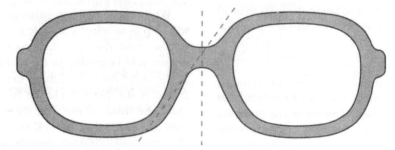

Larger frontal angle

Again, because of the flatness of the nose the frontal angle needs to be larger than an adult frame (more nasal shape). The child's nose has less projection at the bridge.

Ability to shorten temples

Because their heads are relatively small and the length to bend much shorter than an adult, the length of the temples needs to be shorter than the average adult frame (135*mm*). Moreover, it is an advantage if the sides can be shortened, as they can on most metal frames, so that there is not an excessive angle down.

Spring hinges

Given the propensity for children to be rough with their glasses, taking them off with one hand and being hit by basketballs etc, a spring hinge is a definite advantage. Not only will it provide some much needed durability, but it will also help to hold the adjustment longer.

Metal majority

At present most children's frames are metal. Indeed, over 95% of frames dispensed to children are metals. The ability to adjust the pads to meet the criteria above and the fact that metals can now be made in the bright colours of plastic frames has made them an ideal choice.

Many of you will have noticed that the facial features of children are very similar to that of many Asian people. The same criteria apply to the selection of frames to suit an Asian nose. It is also true that metal frames are preferred for fitting an Asian bridge.

When selecting the frame for the child there is one other important consideration that needs to be made. From a safety point of view it is important to make sure that the frames have no sharp edges.

Although an expensive material, titanium is an ideal frame material for children. It is very light and comfortable, holds its shape well and is very durable. Is it too expensive for a children's frame? Many manufacturers don't appear to think so: nor do I. The issues of cost and communication with parents will be discussed later, so we will return to this issue.

Fashion criteria

We should apply the face-shape theory we would use for adults: soft curves for square faces, angular shapes for round faces, a shallow frame for a short face and a deep frame for a long face. We should also make use of colour matching to select a frame that suits the child's skin tones.

While these fashion principles will help us to select a suitable frame for the child, the overriding consideration is to be guided by the wishes of the child. Even if we think that a frame is the perfect choice for a child, the child will not wear them if they are not happy. As well as face shape and colour theory, there is one other important guiding principle for frame selection.

Match width

Choose a frame that matches the width of the child's face, just as you would do with an adult. The frame should coincide as nearly as possible with the width of the face at the temples. Avoid the desire to supply frames that they can 'grow into'. While parents will often select clothes this way, it is not appropriate with spectacles. If the spectacles are too wide it will mean:

1 They will be more easily knocked off the child's face. They will be less stable and could be hit by a glancing blow, or even the child's own hands.

2 There will be compromises made in the optical considerations of the spectacles, like aberrations and thickness. Lenses that are too large will create aberrations near the edge of the lens that would be eliminated by a smaller eyesize. The larger eyesize will also mean thicker, heavier and uglier lenses than necessary.

3 Children will reject oversized frames, Just as they reject oversize clothes. They may put up with oversized school uniforms, to keep their parents happy. They see school clothes as a necessary evil; it is highly unlikely that they would wear them to a social occasion. Their social wardrobe, however, is a different thing. Here they are less likely to be happy with unstylish clothes. Their spectacles fit a social purpose: they are not a part of their uniform.

Some tips on selection

Kids normally know what they like and are very honest. This makes frame selection quite a bit easier. They rarely have preconceived ideas about their image, at least not usually until their early teens. The teens usually have a very definite idea about their image. Once again, though, this can often simplify frame selection.

With younger children (up to about 9), there are a few techniques that will help you to make frame selection easier. Reassure them with comments such as, 'We're going to try everything on that fits you'. This will assure them that you will not miss something out. It doesn't mean that you will try on every frame, since you did limit it to frames that will fit. You can also use terms like 'that looks cool or cute' (relate language to age) and be honest. For the young child you can ask, 'Does this go in the good pile or the bad pile?' This helps to home in on the final choice faster.

The main complicating factor in frame selection is not the child but the parents.

If only the child was present, frame selection in most cases would be relatively simple. Since this is an unlikely situation we need to address the problem of the parent. We will do this shortly.

LENS SELECTION
Technical *criteria*

Lens selection is an extremely important part of paediatric dispensing. As with frame selection, there are some ideal characteristics of lenses for children. The ideal lens should be:

- impact-resistant
- light and comfortable
- able to cut out ultraviolet
- relatively thin
- relatively durable.

Impact-resistant

This is the most important characteristic. As I mentioned earlier, children are rough with their spectacles and themselves. What is worse, other children are often rougher. Children are at considerable risk of injury in the playground, on the sports field, in the backyard and, even in the classroom.

While the odd broken bone or bad bruise may not have any long-term effect, a serious blow to the much more delicate eye could. Vision is a critical sense and the eyes which provide that vision are in need of some protection, especially in childhood.

Light and comfortable

Children will only want to wear something that is comfortable. If spectacles are thick, heavy and uncomfortable, it will be much more difficult to encourage the child to wear them.

Able to cut out ultraviolet

As a community we are much more aware of the detrimental, even dangerous, effects of ultraviolet (UV). We encourage our children to wear sun screen, hats and shirts etc when out in the sun. We are also aware of the effects of UV on eyes. All lenses will provide more protection against UV than wearing no spectacles, but it is certainly a positive feature if the lens absorbs almost all of the incident UV.

Relatively thin

As with weight and comfort, children will be happier wearing spectacles that look nice. No longer can we get away with using large stock lenses for hyperopes, with the resulting thick edges as well as centre thickness. As a hyperope, I can recall with horror the little glass bricks I used to wear as a child.

Relatively durable

Given the roughness of children's behaviour one would hope that lenses would have a reasonable life. Obviously, how long that may be will depend on the individual child. In these circumstances we can not expect too much of the durability of the lenses, and hence the reference to 'relative' durability. By that I mean, relative to the treatment the lenses will receive.

Polycarbonate

Polycarbonate fits the above criteria. It is the lens Superman would wear! Although many other materials meet the last four criteria, polycarbonate is in a class of its own in the first criterion, impact resistance. Indeed, polycarbonate is among the best on the next three criteria, being very light (specific gravity = $1.20g/cm^3$), cutting out almost all solar ultraviolet and being relatively thin (with a relatively high refractive index of $n_d = 1.586$). Today's polycarbonates also perform quite well in durability. Their surface coatings are of similar quality to CR-39 coatings. New coatings are even harder and ideal for children.

DEALING WITH PARENTS

The key to dealing with the concerns of parents is to prioritise the conflicting needs of parents and the child. Many parents will bring with them durability and price as their chief concerns. What may need to be done is to replace these concerns on the parents' list of priorities with things that are more in the interests of the child.

Fashion, comfort and safety are more important to the child than the durability of the spectacles. That does not mean that durability is unimportant, but merely that it does not deserve priority.

Safety is the critical issue

Nothing else deserves higher priority. A dispensing optician has a duty of care to warn parents and children of eye protection. The duty to warn can also be viewed as a duty to inform, to let the patient know the most appropriate lens and frame options.

Take the emphasis out of durability

A child is more likely to wear frames they like than a sturdy, durable frame. Fortunately, in modern frames fashion and durability are not mutually exclusive. This is particularly true of titanium children's frames. In the case of comfort, once again, children will not wear frames that are uncomfortable no matter how solid and long-lasting they might be (after all, they are not paying for them). Again, modern frames are also comfortable.

How long should spectacles last?

Let's consider the issue of durability in more detail. The implication is that the spectacles should be long-lasting. But, how long? And, should children's spectacles last as long as an adult's?

There are two main factors that influence the expected life of spectacles for children. First, children grow rapidly. As with shoes, they will outgrow their frames, usually within a year, certainly no more than two. The spectacles should be changed before they are outgrown. Second, and perhaps even more importantly, no matter how good the quality of the lens surface or coating, the lenses will become scratched after a period of time. Scratched lenses lose their impact resistance. The deeper and more numerous the scratches, the greater the loss of impact resistance. This is not just true of toughened glass as many believe, but also plastic materials including polycarbonate. Of course, polycarbonate has a lot more impact resistance to lose, so a scratched polycarbonate lens is still going to be much more impact-resistant than other materials unscratched. Nevertheless, scratched lenses are an excellent reason to change the spectacles regularly; at least once a year for children.

Yet another reason for replacing spectacles sooner relates to frame standards. British Standard *BS 6625* has two grades for children's frames. According to the standard. Grade B metal for younger children is not expected to last more than one year. This would imply that for younger children, where the growth (and, probably, roughness) is greatest, the spectacles are expected to be changed more frequently than annually.

Treading the fine line between parent and child

Because of the duality of the patient, it is sometimes difficult knowing who to deal with as the primary patient. Try to judge whether the parent or parents are dominant. If they are you should, when speaking to the child, use phrases like, 'You need to like the frame but mum and dad need to like it too: they have to look at you'. Also, have a quiet word with the dominant parent and point out the need for the child to be involved. Explain to them that if the child is involved they are more likely to like their spectacles and so wear them.

Find out what the parents' main concerns are and reassure them that you will steer them in that direction as far as possible. If the parents' wishes are not in the interests of the child (for example, glass lenses), you may need to persuade them into changing their view, using the arguments we have discussed above.

If the parents are OK, speak to the child. This is, of course, the preferred situation but, don't leave the parent entirely out of the picture.

COMMUNICATING WITH KIDS

There are a few tips that can assist you when communicating with kids. Strangely enough, kids like rules, especially young children. So, provide them with simple rules that they can remember, and repeat, such as, 'Use two hands and lift up over your ears'.

Make use of rhymes with young children. For example, 'When they're not on your face, they live in their case'. They will remember these more readily. This particular rhyme also has the advantage of giving the spectacles a personality, something they can relate to.

Use questions, for example, 'Why don't you put your glasses down on their lenses?' The answer often given for this question is that the lenses will get dirty (not scratched). Perhaps this is why so many adults put their spectacle lenses down; they don't even associate that action with scratching the lenses.

Use humour. For example, 'What's the cleaning cloth for? To which they will answer, 'Cleaning your glasses.' Then ask, 'What's your shirt for?' More times than not you will get the same answer, to which you can reply, 'No, it's for wearing.' The message will get through: use the cleaning cloth to clean your glasses, not your clothes. Kids are used to being taught how to clean their teeth by dentists; optical dispensing opticians should teach how to care for their spectacles.

Keep the conversation light, joke with them, have fun.

Also, speak to them at their height —for little children, sit on the floor with the child's parents. They will be more relaxed if you are down in their world and not talking at them from on high, as most adults do.

The kids' corner

If you intend to do a reasonable amount of paediatric dispensing, you may wish to dedicate a certain part of the practice to them. Have a special display designed. It should be colourful and have mirrors at different heights, to cater for the different age groups.

Sit next to the child with the parent behind the child, looking into the mirror with the child. This way the child and the parent can see the child's face at the same time and you will be in a position to select the frames and put them on the child's face.

Have the toy box a little to the side (to amuse siblings). Siblings can be a hindrance. If the toy box is right next to the 'Kids' Corner', they can still distract. You can also distribute puzzles and so forth around the practice to amuse children of adult patients and to help prevent them taking frames off racks. Inquisitive children, however, are inevitable and if you intend to have a paediatric practice you will need to be relaxed about little hands in drawers and racks etc. That does not mean that you don't take steps to prevent it happening.

It is also a good idea to give small gifts to your child patients (balloons, small soft toys). Lollies or sweets can be a bit problematic since many parents are sensitive about their children eating 'rubbish'. You can even give them the former that was used to cut out their lenses, or their old lenses. These are items that their friends at school are unlikely to have! They are a curiosity that they may like to take to school for 'show and tell'.

FACIAL MEASUREMENTS

PDs

Taking PDs can be difficult with children, In the case of older children use the pupillometer as you would with adults. They present no real difficulty.

Younger children, on the other hand, can be a little more difficult. Many may be too young for the pupillometer (too narrow for its range or unable to follow the instructions properly). In such cases, use the PD rule. Try involving the child in the task. Give the child another PD rule to play with and let them take your PD.

For very young children the pupillometer, unfortunately, is not an option. In such cases you will need to use the PD rule and measure from inner to outer canthus. This technique will also work for cases of strabismus (or squint).

Centres

The frames should be chosen so that the centres are as close as possible to geometric centres of the frame. This should also apply to vertical heights of the centres (so that the edge thickness is even all of the way around). You should also use the principal axis/centre of rotation rule so that any aberrations are minimised. If you have selected your frame well, the centres should be on or very near the horizontal centre line. For example, if the pantoscopic tilt were 8°, the pupils should sit about 4 mm above the horizontal centre line of the frame you have chosen. The optical centres will then be on the horizontal centre line.

Bifocals

Some children are prescribed bifocals, usually for convergence problems. If bifocals are prescribed, the segs should be set on pupil centre. While this might seem a bit high compared to normal heights for bifocals, it is considered to be the best place for children. The reason is that, if set any lower, the child would tend to look over the top of the seg. As with fitting bifocals to adults, the easiest way to measure the heights is by premarking the dummy lens.

Summary

Paediatric dispensing can be fun and most certainly rewarding. There are definitely challenges, such as dealing with both parents and child (and possibly even siblings), but the efforts are well worth it. A colleague once said to me that one of his greatest joys as an optical dispenser was putting a new pair of spectacles on a young hyperope or child with strabismus and watching the turned eye straighten up.

If you have a good paediatric practice you can develop patients for life. You should also consider the parents and friends of the children.

12. PRISMATIC EFFECTS

In chapters 9 & 10 we considered plano ophthalmic prisms and the measurement of interpupillary distances and centration distances. We will now look at prisms which form part of a prescription and can be incorporated either by working onto the lens during the grinding process or by decentring the lens.

Fig.12.1 represents a thin plus spherical lens with **O** as the optical centre. A fundamental property of spherical lenses is that incident rays parallel to the optical axis are made to pass through [or to appear to diverge from] an axial point F' known as the *second principal focus*. This evidently requires the rays to undergo different amounts of deviation, according to the distance of the point of incidence from the optical centre. Since deviation is also the characteristic effect of a prism, the action of a lens deviating incident light rays is termed its *prismatic effect*.

Fig.12.1 Prismatic effect of a spherical lens

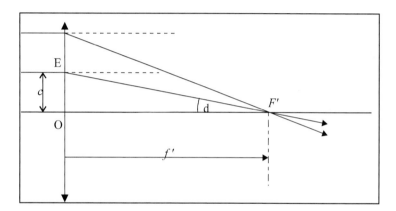

In the diagram above consider the ray incident at the point **E** at a distance **c** [centimetres] from the optical centre. The deviation **d** undergone by the ray is equal to the angle **EF′O**. Hence, the prismatic effect **P** in prism dioptres is $P = 100(c/f')$ if f' is also in centimetres. Finally, since the power F of a thin lens is equal to $100/f'$ where f' is the focal length in centimetres,

$$P = c.F \quad [Prentice's\ Rule]$$

E.g. To find the prismatic effect of a +5.00D lens at a point 5mm [0.5cm] from its optical centre using Prentice's rule we have

$$P = 0.5 \times 5.00 = 2.5\ \Delta\ .$$

As stated previously ophthalmic prisms need to have both magnitude and direction. In order to enable us to state the direction we need to know the direction of the decentred point from the optical centre of the lens in addition to its distance.

Let us consider a –6.00*DS* which has been decentred inwards by 3*mm* in front of a right eye [see Fig.12.2].

Fig.12.2 A –6.00*DS* decentred 3 *mm* in before the right eye

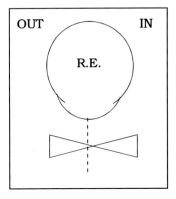

If we think of a minus lens as two prisms with their apexes together and a plus lens as two prisms with their bases together, then we can readily visualise the base directions involved when decentring such lenses. You will see from the diagram above that by decentring the minus lens in before the right eye, we make the eye look through the lens at a point nearer to the outside edge of the lens and consequently the lens will have a base out [180°] prismatic effect. The magnitude can be found as before from Prentice's rule.

$$P = 0.3 \times -6.00 = 1.8\ \Delta$$

Therefore the prismatic effect produced by decentring a –6.00*DS* lens by 3*mm* in before the right eye is 1.8 Δ base OUT.

Fig.12.3   A +8.00 *DS* lens decentred 2.5 *mm* up before the left eye

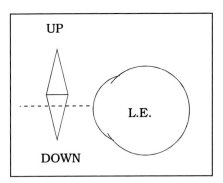

The base of any prismatic effect is always towards the nearest thickest part of the lens from the viewing point.

We can see from Fig.**12**.3 that by decentring a +8.00*DS* upwards in front of a left eye we make the eye look through a point lower down the lens thus producing a base up prismatic effect. As before the exact effect is 0.25 × 8.00 = 2 Δ base UP [90°]

You should have noticed that the base direction is dependent upon the relative position of the eye to the optical centre. In other words we could have worded the above example as 'what is the prismatic effect at the left eye when it looks through a +8.00*DS* lens at a point 2.5*mm* below the optical centre?' The answer is the same.

When dealing with problems involving prisms or prismatic effects you should get into the habit of making a sketch of the lens involved and its position in relation to the eye.

Prismatic effects in sphero-cylindrical lenses

Sphero-cylinders can also be decentred to produce a prescribed prismatic effect. It is worth remembering here that a lens, which is not centred correctly, will produce what may well be an undesired prismatic effect. If the base-apex line of a prescribed prism lies with one of the principal meridians of a sphero-cylinder, then calculations are quite simple. We simply find the prismatic effect for each meridian separately. That is we must apply Prentice's rule to both the axis meridian and the power meridian. However, when we apply Prentice's rule to the axis meridian we will obtain a rather odd result. The prismatic effect in this meridian will be zero. Note then that a prismatic effect can only be created along a meridian, which has power.

E.g. Suppose we are required to calculate the prismatic effect at a point 6*mm* below and 4*mm* in from the centre of a plano/+4.00*DC* × 180 [right eye].

Firstly let us consider the optical cross [Fig.**12**.4]

Fig.12.4

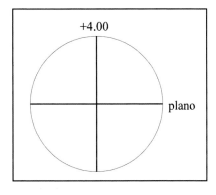

Secondly, calculate the prismatic effect in the power meridian [90°].
$$P = c.F$$
$$= 0.6 \times 4 = 2.4 \; \Delta \; \textbf{[Remember } c \textbf{ is in centimetres]}$$

Since we are below the centre of a plus lens, the direction of the prism base is up. So the prismatic effect 6 *mm* below the centre of a plano/+4.00DC × 180 lens is 2.4 Δ base UP. Since there is no power in the axis meridian, the prismatic effect will be zero. Hence the 2.4 Δ base UP is the complete prismatic effect of our lens.

Let us now consider a slightly more complex lens. Suppose we need to calculate the prismatic effect at a point 8*mm* in and 5 *mm* below from the centre of a right lens of prescription –2.00DS/+6.00DC × 90.

Firstly draw the optical cross diagram.

Fig.12.5

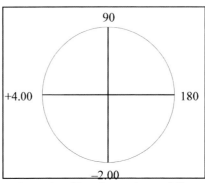

Secondly calculate the prismatic effect in each meridian:

$$P_{90} = c.F \qquad\qquad P_{180} = c.F$$
$$P_{90} = 0.5 \times 2 = 1.0\Delta \qquad\qquad P_{180} = 0.8 \times 4 = 3.2\Delta$$

Since we are in from the centre of a plus lens, the direction of the prism base is out, and since we are below the centre of a minus lens, the direction of the prism base is down. So the prismatic effect 8*mm* below and 5*mm* in from the centre of a right lens –2.00DS/+6.00DC × 90 is 1 Δ base DOWN and 3.2 Δ OUT.

We can if we want compound these prisms into a single resultant as shown in Chapter 9. Using Pythagoras theorem from the triangle **OVR**

$$OR^2 = OV^2 + VR^2 \quad \therefore OR^2 = 1^2 + 3.2^2 = 11.24 \quad \therefore OR = \sqrt{11.24} = 3.35$$

$$\tan V\hat{R}O = OV \div VR = 1 \div 3.2 = 0.3125 \quad \therefore V\hat{R}O = 17.35° \text{ or } 197.35°$$

Cylinders with oblique axes

While cylinders with axes at 90° or 180° are no more difficult than spheres for calculating prismatic effects, cylinders with oblique axes do present more of a problem. In such cases it is possible to determine the prismatic effect at any point on the lens with the use of formulae or by measurement.

The calculation of the prismatic effect at any point on a cylindrical lens with an oblique axis involves the use of a set of formulae. It also requires strict adherence to a set of rules and sign conventions. The notation used in the formulae is as follows and illustrated in Fig.**12.6**.

Sign conventions

F_{sph} = the power of the spherical component of the lens

F_{cyl} = the power of the cylindrical component of the lens

P = the point at which the prismatic effect is to be calculated

x = the horizontal distance from the optical centre [*cm*]

y = the vertical distance from the optical centre [*cm*]

θ = axis of cylinder

H = the horizontal prismatic effect

V = the vertical prismatic effect

Where P is in from the optical centre: x is positive for the right lens and negative for the left lens

P is out from the optical centre: x is negative for the right lens and positive for the left lens

P is up from the optical centre: y is negative

P is down from the optical centre: y is positive

If   H is negative: prism is base to the RIGHT

H is positive: prism is base LEFT

V is negative: prism is base DOWN

V is positive: prism is base UP

The vertical prismatic effect at **P** due to the spherical component of the lens   = yF_{sph}. The horizontal prismatic effect at **P** due to the spherical component of the lens = xF_{sph}. The prismatic effect at **P** due to the cylindrical component of the lens is the product of the perpendicular distance of **P** from the cylinder axis in *cm* and the power of the cylinder [$PR \times F_{cyl}$ in Fig.12.6], the prism base lying along **PR**

Fig.12.6 Prismatic effects at point P

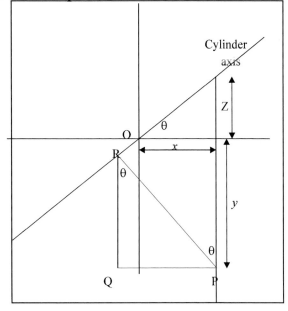

From Fig.12.6 we have:

$$PR = (y + z) \cos \theta$$

where $\quad z = x \tan \theta$

$$\therefore PR = y \cos \theta + x \tan \theta \cos \theta$$
$$= y \cos \theta + x \sin \theta$$

Vertical prismatic effect at P due to cylinder

$$= F_{cyl} RQ$$

$$= F_{cyl} PR \cos \theta$$

$$= F_{cyl} \cos \theta (y \cos \theta + x \sin \theta)$$

Horizontal prismatic effect at P due to cylinder

$$= F_{cyl} QP$$

$$= F_{cyl} PR \sin \theta$$

$$= F_{cyl} \sin \theta (y \cos \theta + x \sin \theta)$$

Adding the effects exerted by the spherical element of the prescription we have:

Total vertical prismatic effect at P:

$$V = -yF_{sph} - F_{cyl} \cos \theta (y \cos \theta - x \sin \theta)$$

Base UP when V is positive
Base DOWN when V is negative

Total horizontal prismatic effect at P:

$$H = -xF_{sph} + F_{cyl} \sin \theta (y \cos \theta - x \sin \theta)$$

Base LEFT when H is positive
Base RIGHT when H is negative

E.g. Calculate the prismatic effect at a point 11 *mm* below and 2½ *mm* inwards from the optical centre of the lens R. +6.00DS/–3.00DC × 140.

We have:

$$F_{sph} = +6 \qquad F_{cyl} = -3$$

$$x = +0.25 \qquad y = +1.1$$

$$\theta = 140$$

$$V = yF_{sph} + F_{cyl}(y \cos^2 \theta + x \sin \theta \cos \theta)$$
$$= (1.1 \times 6) -3 [1.1 \times \cos^2 140 + 0.25 \times \sin 140.\cos 140]$$
$$= 6.6 - 3 [0.6455 \ -0.1231]$$
$$= +5.034\Delta \text{ or } 5.034\Delta \text{ base UP}$$

$$H = xF_{sph} + F_{cyl}(y \sin \theta \cos \theta + x \sin^2 \theta)$$
$$= (0.25 \times 6) -3 [1.1 \times \sin 140.\cos 140 + 0.25 \times \sin^2 140)]$$
$$= 1.5 - 3[-0.5416 + 0.1033]$$
$$= +2.81\Delta \text{ or } 2.81\Delta \text{ base OUT}$$

The above formulae can be transformed to find the vertical and horizontal decentrations (x and y) required to produce a prescribed prism. The same sign convention is used.

We have from the above:

$$V = yF_{sph} + F_{cyl}\left(y\cos^2\theta + x\sin\theta\cos\theta\right)$$

and

$$H = xF_{sph} + F_{cyl}\left(y\sin\theta\cos\theta + x\sin^2\theta\right)$$

which expressions form a pair of simultaneous equations, which can be solved by means of determinants to give:

$$y = \frac{\left(F_{sph} + F_{cyl}\sin^2\theta\right)V - (F_{cyl}\sin\theta\cos\theta)H}{F_{sph}\left(F_{sph} + F_{cyl}\right)}$$

and

$$x = \frac{\left(F_{cyl}\sin\theta\cos\theta\right)V - (F_{sph} + F_{cyl}\cos^2\theta)H}{F_{sph}\left(F_{sph} + F_{cyl}\right)}$$

E.g. Decentre the lens R –2.50DS/+3.00DC × 60 to obtain 4 Δ base IN and 3 Δ base UP.

$$F_{sph} = -2.5 \qquad F_{cyl} = +3$$
$$V = +3 \qquad H = -4$$
$$\theta = 60$$

$$y = \frac{\left(F_{sph} + F_{cyl}\sin^2\theta\right)V - (F_{cyl}\sin\theta\cos\theta)H}{F_{sph}\left(F_{sph} + F_{cyl}\right)}$$

$$= \frac{(-2.5 + 3\sin^2 60)3 - (3\sin 60\cos 60) - 4}{-2.5(-2.5+3)}$$

$$= -3.56cm \text{ downwards}$$

$$x = \frac{\left(F_{cyl}\sin\theta\cos\theta\right)V - (F_{sph} + F_{cyl}\cos^2\theta)H}{F_{sph}\left(F_{sph} + F_{cyl}\right)}$$

$$= \frac{(3\sin 60\cos 60)3 - (-2.5 + 3\cos^2 60) - 4}{-2.5(-2.5+3)}$$

$$= +2.48cm \text{ inwards}$$

The required decentrations are therefore 3.56 *cm* DOWN and 2.48 *cm* IN.

The graphical construction for the above is carried out using the following rules:

1. Construct vertical and horizontal meridians and the principal meridians of the lens.

2. Draw prisms to scale with their bases in the correct directions and construct resultant point Z.

3. Resolve the prisms along the principal meridians of the lens (ZY and ZX) by dropping perpendiculars from Z to the principal meridians.

4. Measure ZY and ZX and calculate the magnitude and direction of the decentrations necessary to produce them (OR and OQ).

5. Compound the decentrations OR and OQ into a single resultant decentration OP and resolve OP into vertical and horizontal components PV and PH.

Fig.12.7   **R –2.50*DS*/+3.00*DC* × 60 to obtain 4 Δ IN and 3 Δ UP.**

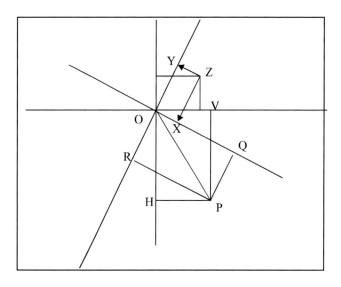

13. BIFOCALS

Introduction

Because of the ageing process of the eye known as *presbyopia,* plus spherical power needs to be added to a distance correction to make near vision possible. The way in which this is done is dependent upon several factors. The type of correction, the hobbies and functional requirements of the patient need to be taken into consideration when deciding upon the solution.

Single vision spectacles for close work can be used to provide the extra plus power, but are often inconvenient. This is where multifocal lenses come in. Multifocal is a term, which can be used to describe any lens, which has more than one portion or area of different power. Although some people take the term to refer to *trifocals* or *progressive* lenses, it also covers *bifocals* as well.

Bifocals provide two prescriptions in the same lens and whilst the majority contain distance and near prescriptions they can of course have any combination of ranges. There seems to be reluctance on the part of some patients to wear bifocals. Whether this is because they are seen as an admission of old age or whether they feel that they "could not get used to bifocals". Many use an alternative such as a half-eye, perhaps to indicate to everyone that "....there is nothing wrong with my eyesight - I only need magnifying lenses to see small print" To me this would not seem to negate the objection to bifocals.

As far as multifocals are concerned, then we have as options, bifocals, trifocals and progressive lenses.

Bifocals and trifocals as their names suggest contain two and three portions respectively of different corrections. Progressive lenses have a main area usually containing a distance correction and an area in which the power of the correction gradually increases until it reaches a point of maximum.

Bifocals mostly contain a distance and a near portion, but can contain any combination of distance, intermediate and near corrections, as required. Trifocals likewise can contain any combination of these three corrections. There are many commercially available types of bifocals, trifocals and progressive lenses in a bewildering assortment of materials. I apologise in advance for the fact that some of the types discussed in this chapter may go out of production for one reason or another, and some others will appear on the scene before the book appears in print. Such is the way of (optical) life.

When discussing bifocals it is difficult to know where to begin as there is such a lot to discuss. Do we list the different styles of which there are hundreds or the types according to method of manufacture? What about their advantages and disadvantages? They could be classified according to their material or availability. I propose to continue from the previous chapter and discuss them according to their main types and give a little more detail as to their manufacture.

Segment specifications

Multifocal segments have developed their own set of dimensions, which we need to examine in order to complete, the picture of frame and lens measurements.

It should be noted that there is a certain amount of confusion relating to these measurements as a result of inconsistent usage. I will try to cover most of these inconsistencies below. The following segment dimensions can be found in figure 13.1.

Fig.13.1 Flat top segment specifications

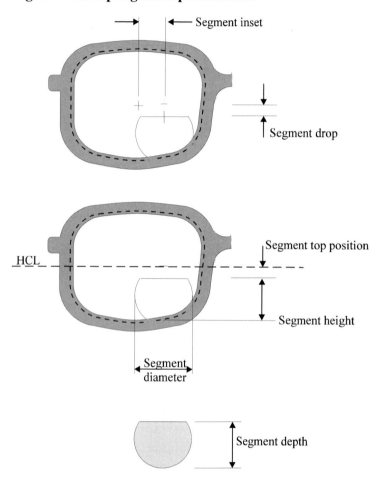

Segment diameter

This is the widest horizontal measurement of the segment. In the case of the D seg this is not the width of the line at the top but, rather, at the widest point. Effectively this is the diameter of the circle if it were a full round seg.

Segment size

This is the segment diameter or width and, in the case of a shaped bifocal, its diameter and its depth.

Segment height

This is the vertical distance from the segment top to a horizontal line tangent to the lens periphery at its lowest point. In the boxing frame measurement, it is the bottom line of the box.

Many interpret the segment height as the distance from the horizontal centre line or datum to the top of the segment, but this is more correctly known as the segment top position.

Segment drop

This is the vertical distance from the segment top to the distance optical centre. Many interpret the segment drop to be the distance from the horizontal centre line to the segment top, but (just as we found with the segment height) this is more correctly known as the segment top position. The segment drop is determined during the surfacing of the back surface. It is set when marking up for the generator.

Segment depth

This is the vertical distance from the segment top to a horizontal line tangent to the segment bottom at its lowest point.

Segment top position

This is the vertical distance from the horizontal centre line to the segment top. As I mentioned above, this is often confused with seg height. A measurement given as a seg height of '3mm below the horizontal centre line' (or more commonly, '3mm below datum') is, more correctly, the seg top position.

Segment inset

This is the horizontal distance between the distance optical centre and segment optical centres (not considering prescribed prism). This is sometimes referred to as the geometric inset. Once again, this is determined when grinding the back surface.

Split bifocals

An early type of bifocal was one described by Benjamin Franklin and which was called a *Franklin* or *split* bifocal. It was made by taking two separate lenses,

cutting them in half, and glazing the distance portion in the upper part of the rim together with the near portion in the lower rim. It has the advantage that both the distance and near optical centres can be located in any desired position. Any combination of corrections can of course be incorporated in the 'lens'. One very useful advantage is that prisms can be incorporated independently in the distance and near portions. The process need not be confined to distance and near corrections, or even to single vision combinations. Split trifocals can be made, either with three straight edged single vision lenses being incorporated, or with one portion being a single vision lens and the other portion some kind of bifocal or progressive lens. The permutations are endless, thus making this altogether a very useful type of lens. Its only real disadvantage is its cosmetic appearance, having a pronounced and visible edge at the points of contact of the component lenses. These edges also attract the dirt and are prone to damage.

Fig.13.2 Franklin Split Bifocal

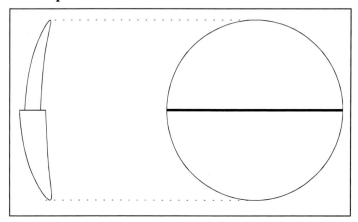

Cemented bifocals

The split lens design was followed by the development of cemented bifocals where a thin convex lens was stuck onto the distance portion. Skilful surfacers could produce extremely thin segments that were known as 'wafers'. These wafers were cemented using Canada Balsam with satisfactory results in most cases. However the cement discoloured with age and the lenses were troublesome when bubbles appeared under the segments. The advantages were similar to those of the split bifocal in that it gave control over the centration of the lenses and provided the contact surfaces were correct prisms etc. could be incorporated. The segment size and shape could also be varied. The disadvantages were exactly the same as with the Franklin bifocal, poor durability and the edges attracted the dirt. I do not know of a currently available lens using this process. There are available *Fresnel* lenses in plus and minus spheres as well as prisms and D25 segments.

Fig.13.3 Cemented Bifocal

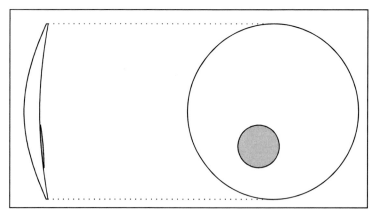

Fused bifocals

Fused bifocals appeared in the early 1900's and utilised two pieces of glass of different refractive indices, the index of the segment being the higher. The originals had round segments but different shapes were later developed. The lens was constructed by the grinding out of a depression in the lower part of the main lens and then fusing a *button* of equal but opposite curvature into the depression. The button was made thicker than the final segment and left proud of the surface of the main lens in order to make it easier to handle. It was then ground and polished to the same curvature as the main lens. If the main lens required an astigmatic correction then this was worked on the opposite surface from that of the segment. The majority of fused bifocals today have the segment on the front surface. If the segment was to be a shaped affair then the button had to be a composite of different shapes and refractive indices in order to obtain the desired result. For example if a flat top segment was required then the button would be made with the lower part of the segment of higher refractive index and the upper part of the same refractive index as the main lens. Thus when the button was fused into the depression the upper part would blend into the main lens [Fig.13.4].

Fig.13.4 Flat top segment [button]

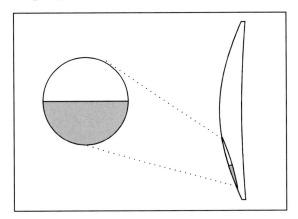

The original fused bifocals used flint glass for the segment and as this had a high dispersion, which resulted in the ensuing chromatic aberration being noticeable around the dividing line of the segment. This effect becomes more pronounced with an increase in segment diameter and also with an increase in the power of the addition as well as when the main lens is negative in power. With the introduction of new glasses of higher refractive index but relatively low dispersion the problem has been considerably reduced and segments of larger diameter are readily available. The use of flat top segments also reduces this effect as well as that of '*image jump*' which we will cover later.

The advantages of fused bifocals are that the segment is inconspicuous and available in a wide variety of shapes. They are not so expensive to make, although I would point out here that the cost of producing a particular type of lens is largely influenced by supply and demand. As mentioned in an earlier chapter the fused 24*mm* round bifocal was the basic type available through the N.H.S. in 1948 and as such there was both a high demand and a controlled price. Although it is still a very useful lens for some cases, it has lessened in popularity and cost has therefore increased proportionally to other lenses. The segment sizes have the limitations described above. The higher refractive index glass used for the segment is softer and as such more prone to damage particularly scratching. It is also not possible to work prisms onto the segments. Although the power of the distance portion of a fused bifocal is not determined until the second side has been surfaced, the reading addition is fixed as soon as the segment side has been finished.

Fig.13.5 Fused Bifocal Segment Shapes

   (a) round segment

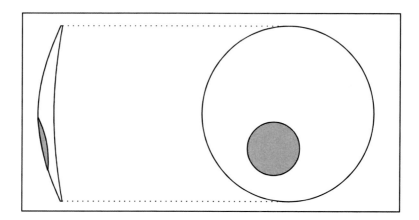

   (b) flat top

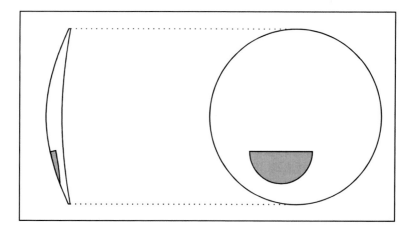

(c) curved top

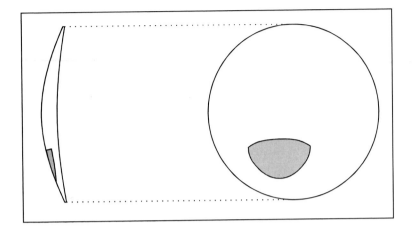

(d) PRO seg

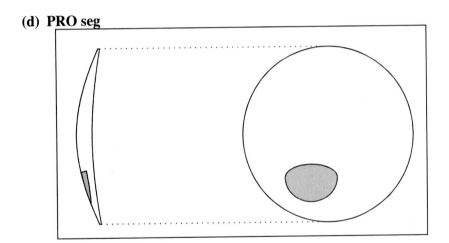

Solid bifocals

Solid bifocals worked from a single piece of glass also appeared in the early part of the century. They originally had the reading portion cut into the distance portion thus producing a pronounced step or ridge. New surfacing machinery was introduced to enable the segment to be produced by a change in curvature thus making the dividing line smooth or *seamless*.

The advantages of solid bifocals are the availability of larger diameter segments, chromatic aberration is negligible, more scratch resistant [glass] and control over the centring of the segment by the use of worked prisms.

There is not such a wide variety of segment shapes in glass but with the advent of plastic lenses the variety has been increased dramatically. The segments can be on either the front or back surface. With non-round segments in the plastic lenses the ridge tends to be very pronounced, particularly with large diameter flat top segments.

Solid Bifocal Segment Shapes
Fig.13.6

   (a) round segment

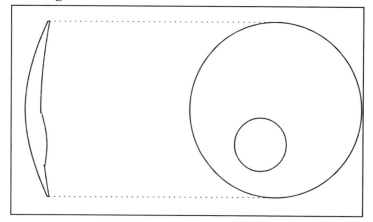

   (b) curved segment

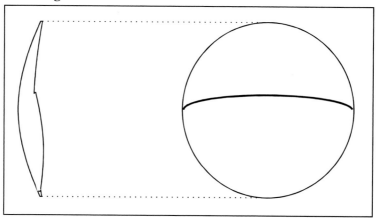

   (c) flat top

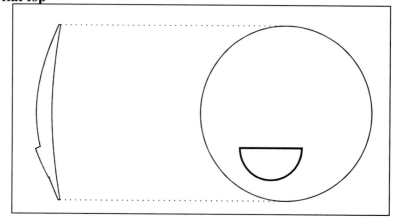

(d) curved top

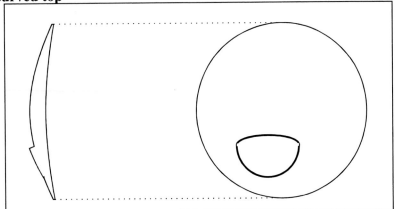

(e) upcurve

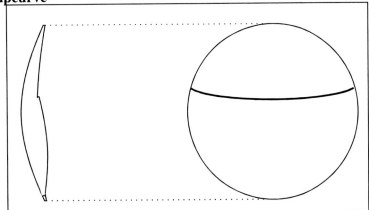

(f) E-type

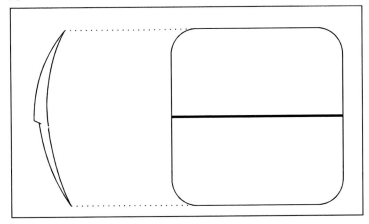

The aforementioned bifocal lenses are currently available in a large variety of shapes, sizes and materials. It is difficult to know how to group them, but here are a few listed.

Fused

> ***Spectacle crown***
> segment on the front surface
> 24 *mm* round
> C25/C28/C32
> D25/D28/D35
> PRO 28 *mm*/32 *mm*
> segment on the back surface
> C25/C28
> ***1.6 index main lens***
> C25/C28
> ***1.7 index main lens***
> D25/C28
> ***1.8 index main lens***
> D25
> ***Photochromic***
> segment on the front surface
> C25/C28
> D25/D28
> segment on the back surface
> C25/C28
> ***Photochromic Shell on High Index Glass***
> ***1.7 & 1.8***
> D25/D28

Solid

> ***Spectacle crown***
> segment on the back surface
> 22 *mm* round
> C25
> 30 *mm*/38 *mm*/45 *mm* round seg.
> E-type
> segment on front surface
> 40 *mm* round
> E-type
> ***1.7 index***
> segment on the back surface
> 22 *mm* round
> ***Upcurves***
> 22 *mm*/38 *mm*/50 *mm*
> ***1.7 index***
> 30 *mm*/38 *mm* round
> ***Photochromic***
> segment on back

30 *mm*/38 *mm* round
segment on front
E-type
CR39
segment on front surface
22 *mm*/24 *mm*/25 *mm*/28 *mm*/38 *mm*/45 *mm* round
D25/D28/D35/D40
C25/C26/C28/C40
E-type

In addition many of the above CR39 bifocals are available with the main portion of the lens in aspheric form.

In an ideal world bifocals would satisfy a number of mechanical, cosmetic and optical conditions.

- The lenses would be no heavier than single vision lenses and have an inconspicuous dividing line.
- The near portion would provide vision as clear as the distance portion.
- There should be no sudden change in prismatic effect at the top of the segment.
- The differential prismatic effect at the near visual points should be within acceptable limits.

Unfortunately it is not an ideal world and, as such, each lens design must of necessity be a compromise.

Measuring heights

We know how to centre bifocals horizontally, having measured the PD. Ideally we will have measured the monocular CDs with the pupillometer and now need to work out where to place the centres vertically.

There are quite a few ways in which the measurements can be taken. We will compare three methods below.

Method 1

1 Adjust the frame so that it is its final fitting.

2 Measure the monocular CDs.

3 Mark the horizontal centre line on the dummy lenses of the frame and draw a vertical line at the monocular PDs, marking off each *2mm* above and below the HCL. Your lenses will look like those in Figure 13.7.

4 Now, with your head and your patient's head at the same level and the patient looking straight ahead with their head in normal posture, note the point which is level with the bottom lid. Ideally, you should be sitting on an adjustable stool

so that you can ensure that you and your patient are at the same height. Take a glance into the wall mirrors to check your positioning.

5 As a double-check, it is wise to then engage your patient in conversation and continue to note the relevant marking—if a patient feels they are being measured their head position is unlikely to be natural. If you are just chatting to them, though, they will not realise that you are taking a measurement.

Fig.13.7 Pre-marking the dummy lenses

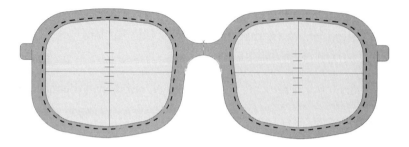

Method 2

1 Adjust the frame so that it is in its final fitting.

2 Measure the PD (preferably monocular).

3 Place the frame with the dummy lenses onto the patient.
With your head at the same level as your patient's, place a dot with a marking pen on the point level with the lid. The patient should be looking across the room with their head in their normal posture.

4 Once again, check the measurement by chatting to the patient (their head position is unlikely to be natural if you are approaching them, armed with a pen). If you use this method, make sure your dots are precise.

Method 3

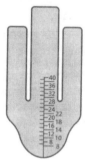

This is the same as method 1 with the exception that inserts are put into the frame instead of the dummy lenses. There is no need, of course, to mark the inserts since they have a millimetre scale which can be used to line up with the lower lid. The inserts are shown in Figure 13.8.

Figure 13.8 Height inserts

Comparison of the methods

Methods 1 and 3 have a distinct advantage over method 2. Since you are not approaching the patient's face with a pen, they are more likely to be natural. It is also much easier for you to simply observe the markings rather that trying the difficult procedure of placing a precise dot on a transparent dummy lens. Moreover, with method 2, if the dots are not in the correct position you need to re-dot the lenses. This is not necessary with methods 1 and 3.

Recommended bifocal heights *Small round seg (24mm seg)*

The small round seg is generally positioned level with the top of the patient's lower lid (see Figure 13.9). This lens is best suited for someone who is not a devoted reader but needs to read for short periods of time. Although it is important not to interfere with their more important distance vision, care must be taken not to set the segs too low. The eyes must drop about *6mm* into the segs to achieve a reasonable reading width.

Fig.13.9 Small round seg   **Fig.13.10 Flat-top bifocals**

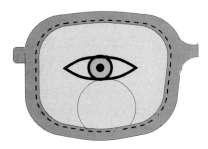 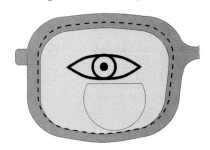

Flat-top bifocals (25 mm seg)

The standard height for flat-top bifocals is *2mm* below the top of the lower lid (that is, *2mm* below the round seg). This seg is now the preferred 'all-rounder' and is suited to someone who is a regular reader. Since a wide reading width is achieved immediately, the seg can be set a little lower than the round seg.

Setting at non-standard positions

The above positions assume normal, everyday use and an 'average' patient. There are cases, however, where the segs should not be set in the standard position.

Posture

If the patient is stooped or has an exceptionally erect stance, the standard height may interfere with their distant or near viewing. For example, a person with an erect stance, head held back, would need their segs set lower than normal to ensure that the segs did not interfere with their distance vision. A person with a stoop, on the other hand, would need the segs set higher to ensure that they had useful vision through the segs.

Vocation

An occupation or hobby that requires either more distance vision or more near vision would necessitate an adjustment to the seg heights. For example, a truck or bus driver would be more concerned with distance vision, especially given their position (high up and very near the front of the cabin) and so their segs should be set lower than normal. An architect or writer, on the other hand, would need their segs set higher.

Previous position

We should consider how they have worn their segs before and how comfortable they were. For example, if they had been wearing their segs at the standard position and were uncomfortable, the new seg positions would have to be non-standard.

On the other hand, if they had been wearing their previous pair at a non-standard position and were very comfortable, logic requires that the new segs be made up non-standard.

Addition

Although this has minimum effect on heights, the add affects the inset required. If an intermediate addition is ordered for, say, reading music, the inset should be set according to the working distance. The pupillometer allows for the near CD to be measured for any working distance.

So if these intermediate bifocals were ordered for reading music, the segs would also need to be set higher in order to read the music, which might be on a stand some distance from the musician, but for piano etc, it is directly in front and only about 50*cm* away.

Occupational bifocals

Occupational bifocals (such as the large round seg, the large flat-top and the Executive) are generally positioned according to need, with the seg often set higher than the standard heights mentioned above: the vocation criterion for fitting mentioned above applies to all of them. The method of determining the heights is still the same, however, with your preferred method for measuring the bifocal heights working equally as well for occupational bifocals. However, consideration must be given to the patient's position. Ask them if the lenses are to be used for some specific purpose such as a computer, switchboard or control panel which may be above eye level.

You might try simulating their working (or playing) position after you have determined the heights. Draw the segs on the dummy lenses with a dark felt-tipped pen and while simulating the working environment have your patient look through the dummy lenses to see the position of the 'segs'. Given the number of presbyopes who play golf or lawn bowls, it might be worthwhile having a golf ball, a driver and an iron for the golfer to simulate addressing the ball, and a bowl for the bowler to hold.

Minimum depths

As with progressives, we need to ensure that the frame we select allows for a reasonable seg depth. While progressive lens manufacturers indicate the minimum depth from the fitting cross to the bottom of the frame, bifocal and trifocal manufacturers do not. It is generally advisable, however, to ensure that there is at least 15*mm* between the seg to and the bottom of the frame (except in cases such as the 'golf' or sportsman bifocal)

The problem with bifocal segment inset involves making the eyes look through the centres of the segments when fixating a point on the median line at the requisite working distance. When this is achieved the two fields of view will coincide, assuming the lens powers are equal. Fig.13.11 indicates the solution and Tables 13.1 and 13.2 list the results using the paraxial approximation:

$$\text{inset} = p\left[\frac{L}{L+F-S}\right]$$

where *p* is the semi-PD, measured for each eye in *mm*, $S = l/s = 1/0.027 = 37D$, and *L* is the object vergence corresponding to the distance stated in the tables.

Rodenstock produce their 22*mm* segment aspheric bifocal Perfastar with a standard 4*mm* inset, although they will make them with 3*mm* and 5*mm* insets to order. It should be obvious from the tables that for high powered lenses the usual method of dividing by two the difference between distance PD and near CD in order to arrive at the inset is not always appropriate.

Fig.13.11 Determination of the bifocal inset to make the reading portion fields coincide.

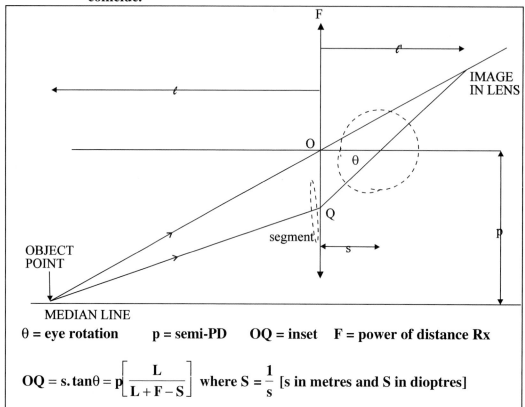

θ = eye rotation   p = semi-PD   OQ = inset   F = power of distance Rx

$$OQ = s.\tan\theta = p\left[\frac{L}{L+F-S}\right] \text{ where } S = \frac{1}{s} \text{ [s in metres and S in dioptres]}$$

Table 13.1 Bifocal inset as a function of object distance, semi-PD and plus distance Rx [values rounded to the nearest half-millimetre]

Semi-PD	Distance Rx	Working distance [cm]			
		25	33	40	50
30	+10.00	4.0	3.0	2.5	2.5
	+12.00	4.0	3.0	2.5	2.5
	+14.00	4.5	3.5	3.0	2.5
	+16.00	5.0	4.0	3.0	2.5
32.5	+10.00	4.0	3.0	3.0	2.5
	+12.00	4.5	3.5	3.0	2.5
	+14.00	5.0	4.0	3.0	2.5
	+16.00	5.0	4.0	3.5	3.0
35	+10.00	4.5	3.5	3.0	2.5
	+12.00	5.0	4.0	3.0	2.5
	+14.00	5.0	4.0	3.5	3.0
	+16.00	5.5	4.5	4.0	3.0

Table 13.2 Bifocal inset as a function of object distance, semi-PD and minus distance Rx [values rounded to the nearest half-millimetre]

Semi-PD	Distance Rx	Working distance [cm]			
		25	33	40	50
30	−10.00	2.5	2.0	1.5	1.0
	−12.00	2.0	2.0	1.5	1.0
	−14.00	2.0	1.5	1.5	1.0
	−16.00	2.0	1.5	1.5	1.0
32.5	−10.00	2.5	2.0	1.5	1.0
	−12.00	2.5	2.0	1.5	1.0
	−14.00	2.5	2.0	1.5	1.0
	−16.00	2.0	1.5	1.5	1.0
35	−10.00	2.5	2.0	2.0	1.5
	−12.00	2.5	2.0	1.5	1.5
	−14.00	2.5	2.0	1.5	1.5
	−16.00	2.5	2.0	1.5	1.5

Prismatic effects

These can be calculated in almost exactly the same way as with single vision lenses as discussed in chapter 11, the only difference being that we must take the effects of the segment into consideration.

E.g. Calculate the prismatic effect at the near visual point situated $11mm$ below and $2\frac{1}{2}$ *mm* inwards from the distance optical centre of the lens:

R −6.00DS/+3.00DC×140 Add +1.50DS. The segment to be *2mm* below and *2mm* inset. We will consider segments of *22mm* round, *38mm* round and D25.

The prismatic effect at the near visual point for the distance portion only can be calculated as follows.
We have:

$$F_{sph} = -6 \quad F_{cyl} = +3 \quad x = +0.25 \quad y = +1.1 \quad \theta = 140$$
$$V = yF_{sph} + F_{cyl}\left(y\cos^2\theta + x\sin\theta\cos\theta\right)$$
$$= (1.1 \times -6) +3\,[1.1\cos^2 140 + 0.25\sin 140\cos 140]$$
$$= -5.03\Delta \text{ or } 5.034\Delta \text{ base DOWN}$$
$$H = xF_{sph} + F_{cyl}\left(y\sin\theta\cos\theta + x\sin^2\theta\right)$$
$$= (0.25 \times -6) +3\,[1.1\sin 140\cos 140 + 0.25\sin^2 140]$$
$$= -2.81\Delta \text{ or } 2.81\Delta \text{ base IN}$$

Fig.13.12

    (a) 22 *mm* round

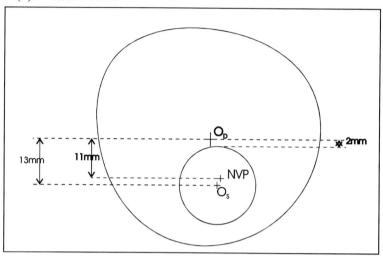

For the *22mm* round segment the centre of the seg is *13mm* below and *2mm* in from the distance optical centre [O_D]. It is therefore *2mm* down and ½*mm* out from the NVP. Using Prentice's rule we get:

$$P_v = c_v F_v = 0.2 \times 1.5 = 0.3\Delta \text{ base DOWN}$$

$$P_h = c_h F_h = 0.05 \times 1.5 = 0.075\Delta \text{ base OUT}$$

    (b) 38 *mm* round

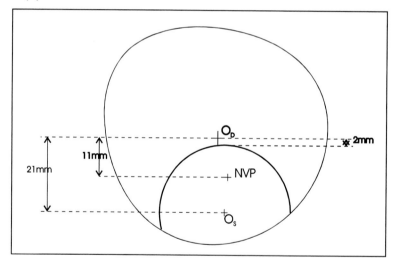

For the *38mm* round segment the centre of the seg is *21mm* below and *2mm* in from the distance optical centre [O_D]. It is therefore *10mm* down and ½*mm* out from the NVP. Again using Prentice's rule:

$$P_v = c_v F_v = 1 \times 1.5 = 1.5\Delta \text{ base DOWN}$$

$$P_h = c_h F_h = 0.05 \times 1.5 = 0.075\Delta \text{ base OUT}$$

(c) D25 seg

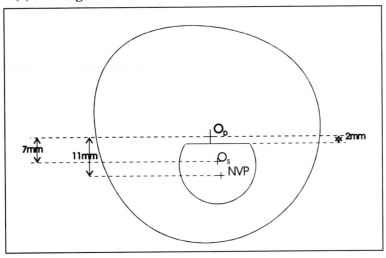

For the D25 segment bifocal the seg is *7mm* below and *2mm* in from the distance optical centre [O$_D$]. This makes its centre *4mm* above and *½mm* out from the NVP. From Prentice's rule:

$$P_v = c_v F_v = 0.4 \times 1.5 = 0.6\Delta \text{ base UP}$$
$$P_h = c_h F_h = 0.05 \times 1.5 = 0.075\Delta \text{ base OUT}$$

<u>Summary</u>

		Vertical	Horizontal
22 *mm*	D	5.03 Δ DOWN	2.81 Δ IN
	seg	0.30 Δ DOWN	0.075 Δ OUT
	TOTAL	5.33 Δ DOWN	2.78 Δ IN
38 *mm*	D	5.03 Δ DOWN	2.81 Δ IN
	seg	1.50 Δ DOWN	0.075 Δ OUT
	TOTAL	6.53 Δ DOWN	2.735 Δ IN
D25	D	5.03 Δ DOWN	2.81 Δ IN
	seg	0.60 Δ UP	0.075 Δ OUT
	TOTAL	4.43 Δ DOWN	2.735 Δ IN

Image Jump

As can be seen from the above calculations when the wearer lowers his gaze away from the optical centre of the lens he experiences an increasing prismatic effect the farther from the optical centre the eyes travel. The segment also produces its own prismatic effect, the value of which is dependent upon the location of the segment optical centre. When the gaze crosses the top of the segment, the prism induced by the distance portion is suddenly changed by the amount of prism induced by the segment portion. This abrupt change in prismatic effect causes objects to be suddenly displaced from the position they just appeared to have when viewed through the distance portion of the lens.

This sudden displacement of the image as the bifocal line is crossed is known as *Image Jump.* <u>The amount of image jump for a given type of bifocal is</u> **independent** <u>of the</u> **distance** <u>portion</u> and can be calculated using Prentice's rule. If we consider the same three types again we have:

$$22mm \text{ round} \quad P = cF = 1.1 \times 1.5 = 1.65\Delta$$
$$38mm \text{ round} \quad P = cF = 1.9 \times 1.5 = 2.85\Delta$$
$$D25 \text{ seg} \qquad P = cF = 0.5 \times 1.5 = 0.75\Delta$$

With any flat top bifocal where the optical centre of the segment coincides with the top then there will of course be no image jump.

14. TRIFOCALS

Introduction

Around the ripe old age of 55 years the reading addition required will have increased to approximately +2.00*D*. This means that the depth of field will have decreased with the result, that whilst the near vision prescription will be fine for small detail, problems will be experienced with visual tasks between 40 and 80*cm*. A lens of about half the dioptric power of the near addition will be required. One way of utilising this is in the form of a *trifocal*.

As with bifocals, trifocals can take various forms, although for a variety of reasons, not so many. Because many people do not relish the thought of coping with two different lenses in one, many more cannot contemplate three in one. The N.H.S. didn't cater for the visual needs of the 'middle-aged' by providing trifocals. These are two of the reasons for trifocals not catching on in large numbers. I suspect that the fact that opticians did not suggest them was another. With the invention of varifocal lenses they have tended to remain in the background, only used by those already wearing them and those with special vocational needs which cannot be satisfied with other forms of lens, and of course varifocal failures.

Trifocals are made in crown glass, photochromic glass and CR39. Below are listed some of the currently available types.

Fused

spectacle crown
segment on the front surface
C28
D25/D28/D35
Double D25
Photochromic
S725
segment on the back surface
C725/C828

Solid

spectacle crown
E-type
CR39
25 *mm* round
C28/C40
D25/D28/D35
S728
E-type
E-D

The intermediate addition is 50% of the near addition in most trifocals. The above types can of course be extended by combining single vision with bifocal lenses using the split method.

Fig.14.1 Trifocals
   (a) round seg

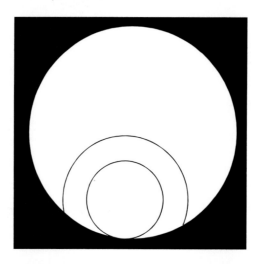

   (b) flat top

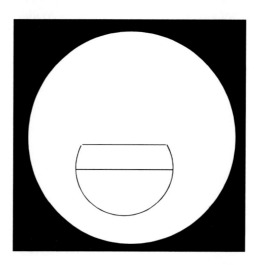

   (c) curved top

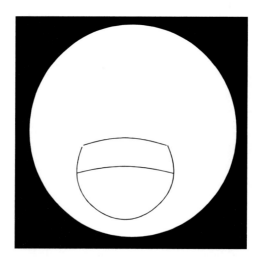

(d) E-type

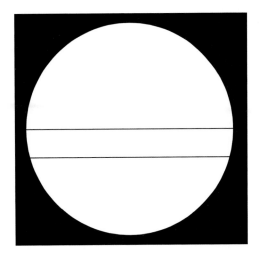

(e) E-D

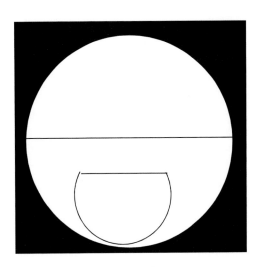

(f) Double D

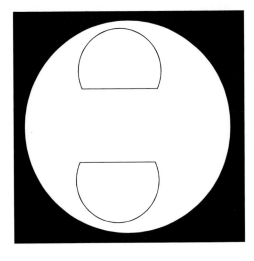

(g) Double curved

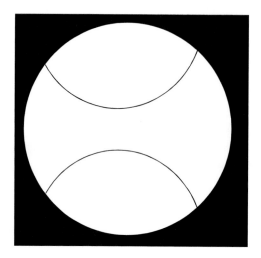

Fitting Trifocals

Trifocals are generally fitted about *2mm* below the bottom of the pupil. This ensures that distance vision is not interfered with too much, but still provides enough depth for the reading and intermediate segments. As with bifocals, trifocals may be set at a non-standard height, depending on the patient's requirements.

The type of trifocal selected and the heights the segs are set at depend largely on the intermediate vision demands of the patient. In cases such as computer operators, card players, and musicians, where the intermediate fields needs to be large, a trifocal with a large intermediate segment set high is most appropriate. If, on the other hand, the intermediate vision is not a major part of the patient's visual needs, a smaller trifocal such as the flat-top trifocal would suffice.

As with bifocals, there are occupational trifocals. The most obvious of these is the Librarian trifocal, so named because it is designed for occupations such as librarian. Given that it has an intermediate seg at the top and a reading seg at the bottom setting the heights can be tricky. The bottom seg can normally be set at the usual position for a flat-top or slightly higher. The important thing to remember is that the segs should not be directly in front of the pupil when the patient is looking straight ahead.

15. PROGRESSIVE LENSES

Introduction

The first commercially available varifocal lens was introduced by Essel in the early 1960s. There have been considerable improvements in both design and production technology, and today there are many different designs of progressive lens available in different types of glass as well as plastic, from which the dispenser can choose.

There are four areas of the lens which perform specific functions, and it is in the size, positioning and treatment of these zones that the different designs of progressive lenses vary. These areas and their functions can be listed as follows.

1. The upper portion designed to provide maximum visual acuity for unimpaired distance viewing.

2. The lower portion designed for any visual task in the near range.

3. A corridor with a progressive power which provides a continuous change of power from distance to near.

4. Temporal and nasal peripheral portions which occupy the remaining areas of the lens.

It is the manner in which these individual parameters are correlated that gives any design of progressive lens its individual character.

The distance area in early designs was usually spherical but second generation lenses have tended towards aspherical surfaces which will assist in blending the distance power into the progressive curve. The reading portion may be large or small, high or low and the lens selected should be the one most suited to the patient's visual needs in the near range.

It is the geometry of the progressive corridor and the peripheral areas which most often affects the performance or acceptance of the lens. The progressive corridor can be fully corrected for surface aberrational astigmatism only along its centre line, and the further we move to the side of this line, the greater will be the aberration. Many people feel that the amount of surface aberrational astigmatism is less important than its direction and that a reasonable amount is tolerable when its axis is horizontal or vertical; when it is oblique an unacceptable amount of 'skew' distortion is produced.

The advantages of progressive lenses are:

- The transition from distance to near vision areas is invisible.

- The cosmetic appearance is the same as a single vision lens.

- With correct fitting of the lens, an acceptable acuity can be obtained at distance, intermediate and near ranges.

- There is no image jump.

Some of the disadvantages are:

- There are areas of surface aberrational astigmatism which result in blur.

- There may be a longer adaptation period than with bifocals.

- More head movement is required during adaptation in order to locate the correct power area.

- The length of the progression zone requires that the eyes must be lowered over a longer distance to look from far to near objects than with conventional downcurve bifocals.

Comparison of the different designs is not an easy task. Let us look at some of the test methods which have been devised.

1. *Schematic sketches*. - This is the over-simplified drawing which shows the basic design philosophy the designer was aiming at but gives no indication of what he has done with the 'naughty bits'.

2. *Grid pattern photography*. - Sometimes a wire mesh is used, or more popularly, the Raster Dot Printing screen and these are photographed through the progressive lens. This will show the basic design outline of the lens. Whilst skew and other distortion are shown up, it gives little indication or otherwise of the wearabilty of the lens.

3. *Vector plot*. - A most useful source of information as it is compiled from computerised measurements of astigmatism taken by scanning the entire surface of the lens. The plots indicate both the amount and the direction of surface aberrational astigmatism.

4. *Astigmatic contour plot*. - This is a sort of weather map in which lines of 'iso-cylinders' of similar amounts of astigmatism are joined together.

5. *Power plot graphs*. - In this method the dioptric power distribution is scanned along specific lines and the values plotted on graphs. The power may be measured on an ordinary focimeter equipped with a type of lens holder which allows the lens to swing across the focimeter aperture, thus representing the refractive power as it

would be perceived by the eye. the reading profile shows the rate of power increase along the progressive corridor.

Figure 15.1 illustrates what these comparisons look like.

Fig.15.1

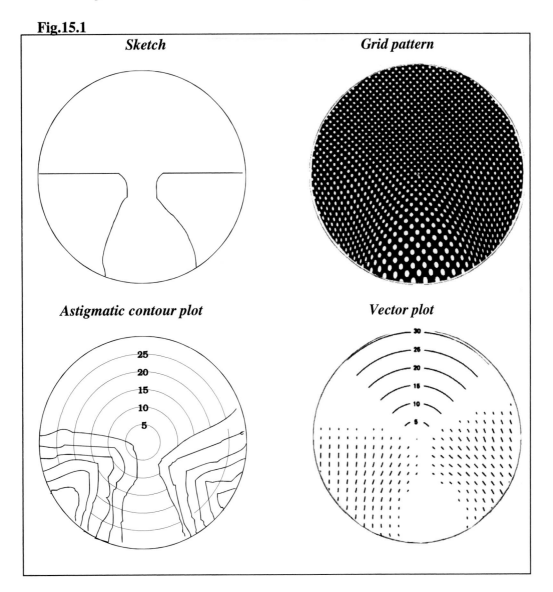

The amount of surface aberrational astigmatism and its distribution across the surface of the progressive lens will determine whether the lens is classified as either hard or soft design.

Hard design lenses are where the surface aberrational astigmatism is confined to the nasal and temporal areas, leaving the distance area aberration free. The progressive zone in such lenses is usually narrow with a comparatively wide reading area. As a result of this hard design lenses are probably more suited to prolonged near vision work with only occasional intermediate use. Current lenses which can be classified as hard design are:- *Elegance, Graduate, Line Free, Truvision A3, Unison S and Visiomild.*

Soft design lenses on the other hand allow for aberrational astigmatism to extend into the distance area which has the effect of reducing the overall strength of the astigmatism but does produce peripheral blurring. At the same time the progressive corridor is wider and a corresponding narrowing of the reading area occurs. This leads to them being more suited to greater intermediate use such as with VDUs. Current lenses which can be classified as soft design are:- *Gradal HS, Gradal 3, Hoyalux 3, Progressiv R, Progressiv S, Truvision Omni, Varilux, VMD and XL.*

The strength of the reading addition has an effect on the width of the reading area in that the greater the add the narrower the reading area becomes. Figure 15.2 illustrates the astigmatic contour plots for several different progressive lenses. The most recent development in progressive lenses has been the use of twelve separate designs, one for each of the adds from 0.75 to 3.50. This is utilised in Essilor's VMD in which unlike other designs the power of the add goes on increasing beyond the centre of the near checking circle.

Fig.15.2

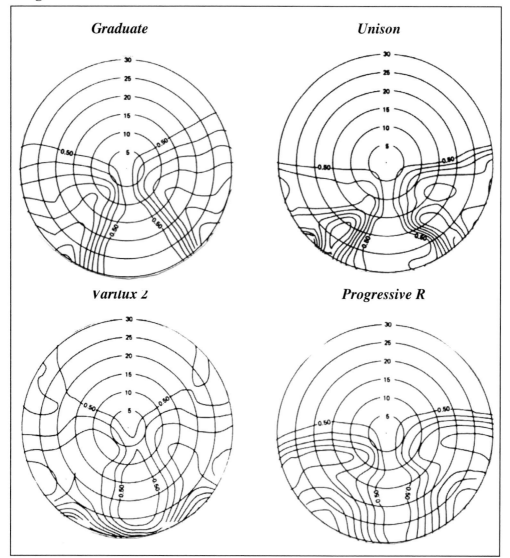

Measuring heights

The standard height for progressive lenses is the centre of the pupil—that is, the fitting cross should line up with the centre of the pupil when the patient is looking into the distance.

Fig.15.3 Fitting progressive lenses

Progressive fitting cross
(pupil centre)

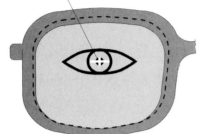

Fitting is an area where there is some considerable argument among dispensers, optometrists and manufacturers. More than one method will do the job: indeed, even the manufacturers are divided in their views on fitting. We will examine a number of methods and compare their advantages and disadvantages.

It is true that some methods will take a little longer (not a lot) but they should not be dismissed on this basis. Care is an important aspect in fitting lenses but the appearance of care can be even more important. Patients will judge on their perceptions.

Method 1

1 Adjust the frame so that it is in its final fitting.

2 Measure the monocular PDs with the pupillometer.

3 Mark the horizontal centre line on the dummy lenses of the frame and draw a vertical line at the monocular PDs, marking off each *2mm* above and below HCL with a fine-tipped pen. A parallel rule is useful for this.

4 Now, with your head and your patient's head at the same level, note the point that is level with the centre of the pupil. You can look into the wall mirrors to help ensure that your heights are the same. Ideally, you should be sitting on an adjustable stool.

5 Check your measurement by engaging your patient in conversation and continuing to note the relevant marking.

6 Now, place the manufacturer's 'eyepoint' gauges on the lenses with the distance circle around the fitting cross you have marked after step 5. If your manufacturer does not produce these gauges (don't confuse them with checking masks), draw a small circle around the fitting cross and another around the top of the near checking circle.

7 Place a mirror, with a circle or cross on it, on the desk between you and your patient. Ask the patient to sit in their 'normal' position and look down at the mirror as though reading. With your right eye look down into the circle. You should see the patient's right eye in the middle of the reading circle in the

eyepoint gauge (likewise, with your left eye and your patient's left eye). Some manufacturers, such as Hoya and Rodenstock, have produced illuminated mirrors for this purpose.

8 If you do not see the reflection of your patient's eyes as described in the above step, move the eyepoint gauges until you do.

9 Order the lens position according to your final positioning of the eyepoint gauges.

Method 2

1 Adjust the frame so that it is in its final fitting.

2 Measure the monocular PDs with the pupillometer.

3 Mark the horizontal centre line on the dummy lenses of the frame and draw a vertical line at the monocular PDs, marking off each *2mm* above and below the HCL with a fine-tipped pen. A parallel rule is useful for this.

4 Now, with your head and your patient's head at the same level, note the point that is level with the centre of the pupil. You can look into the wall mirrors to help ensure that your heights are the same. Ideally, you should be sitting on an adjustable stool.

5 Check your measurement by engaging your patient in conversation and continuing to note the relevant marking.

6 Order the lens position according to your monocular PDs and the heights according to the final positioning of the markings.

Method 3

1 Adjust the frame so that it is in its final fitting.

2 Measure the monocular near CDs with the pupillometer.

3 Mark the horizontal centre line on the dummy lenses of the frame and draw a vertical line at the monocular PDs, marking off each *2mm* above and below the HCL with a fine-tipped pen. A parallel rule is useful for this.

4 Now, with your head and your patient's head at the same level, note the point that is level with the centre of the pupil. You can look into the wall mirrors to help ensure that your heights are the same. Ideally, you should be sitting on an adjustable stool.

5 Check your measurement by engaging your patient in conversation and continuing to note the relevant marking.

6 Order the lens position by adding 2.5*mm* to your monocular near CDs and the heights according to the final positioning of the markings. (This method assumes there is a 2.5*mm* inset created by the manufacturer. Some manufacturers may have a smaller inset—for example, the new AO compact inset varies with power.)

Method 4

1 Adjust the frame so that it is in its final fitting.

2 Measure the monocular PDs (preferably with the pupillometer).

3 Place the frame with the dummy lenses onto the patient. With your head at the same level as your patient's place a dot with a marking pen on the point level with the centre of the pupil. Some people use this to determine the monocular PDs (thus eliminating step 2), although a pupillometer is more likely to give an accurate PD.

4 Check your measurement by engaging your patient in conversation and continuing to note the relevant marking.

5 Order the lenses according to the heights of the dots.

Comparison of the methods

Accuracy

There is likely to be some argument over which is the most accurate. However, the more time that is taken and the greater the built-in checks, the more likely the result will be accurate. Moreover, the fitting position must be related to the wearer's natural posture. The patient cannot 'be natural' if told to be, nor will they be natural if someone is dotting their lenses with a pen. Consider these implications in your choice of a method to adopt. Remember too, that the pupillometer is measuring the distance between the visual axes and not merely the distance between the pupil centres.

Appearance

The measurement must not only be accurate, it must be seen to be accurate. Remember, the patient has just been tested by the optometrist or ophthalmologist with the latest equipment: refractor heads, non-contact tonometers, slit lamps etc. They are unlikely to be impressed by a wooden stick and a felt-tipped pen, especially if they're paying for the lenses but pay nothing for the eye test. They will be expecting considerable care on the part of the optical dispenser when measuring up for these expensive, latest-technology lenses. If your preference is for the pen and ruler, make sure that you appear to be taking care and not rushing the measurement (it goes without saying that you are taking care).

Time

There is no doubt that method 4 is the fastest, but not by a significant margin. With practice, all methods can be done efficiently.

Ease

Some might argue that method 4 is the easiest, but for those who find it difficult to steady their hands, the methods in which the dummy lens is pre-marked are easier.

Other factors to consider

Measuring position

The ideal position for measuring heights is with the patient in a reasonably comfortable (but not lounge) chair. You should be seated on an adjustable stool so that you can adjust your height to suit your patient. Use the wall mirrors to help ensure that you are on the same level. There are plenty of horizontal visual clues to help you do this, such as the frame racks.

You may wish to confirm the setting while standing but it is not advisable to take the measurement this way. It is unlikely that all of your patients will be your height and so your measurements are likely to be out. Of course you can squat down a little for shorter people, but holding that position while you make the measurement is not easy or advisable for your health. Also, when you are double-checking the heights the patient will be aware that you are taking a measurement, given your rather unusual stance. Unless you stand on a box, taller people are even more of a problem!

Comparing the near and distance methods

Method 1 is a 'near' method, based on the principle that you get the near right and the distance will look after itself. It is based on the premise that the near and intermediate are the most restricted zones and so it is critical that we get them right. The advantage of the near method is that it will find those who hold their reading material to one side. It will also pick up people with a convergence problem.

In most cases the near and distance methods will give you the same result but there are the few cases that the near method picks up that the distance method may not.

Summary

Most of the methods will work well most of the time, assuming they are carried out correctly. When choosing your method— and it may not even be one of the four above (it might be a mixture of two of them, for example)—don't just consider speed and convenience.

You may not like my preferred method or you may simply prefer your current method, but is it not worth trying a new method? To quote Franklin D Roosevelt (speaking on the US economy), 'It is common sense to take a method and try it. If it fails, admit it frankly and try another. But above all, try something.'

16. LENS MEDIA

With the gradual demise of the National Health Service in the optical arena there has been a dramatic increase in the use of plastics lenses. The last five years have shown the most rapid increase. Adding to this change in dispensing status has been the proliferation of mid-index and high-index plastics materials. [see table 16.3 on page 88]

Together with higher V-values, these lenses have given rise to a real reduction in the weight of fifty percent on crown glass lenses. Minus CR39 lenses cannot be made with a centre thickness of less than 1.8*mm*, but mid-index plastics approximate to 1.5*mm* and the high-index lenses can be as low as 1.0*mm*.

Where two lenses are identical in form and refractive index, but have different specific gravities, then the lens with the lower specific gravity will result in the lighter lens.

When dispensing lenses the most common demands made are that they should be both as thin as possible and also as light as possible. The main properties of interest to the dispensing optician are refractive index, V-value and specific gravity. The thickness of the lens is controlled by the refractive index. V-values affect off axis performance and specific gravity affects the weight.

If the form and power of two lenses are similar, together with the centre substance, then it can be assumed that the lens having the higher refractive index will be the thinner. From a cosmetic standpoint then minus lenses show the greatest benefit. Relative curvature is useful to be able to predict a saving in edge thickness with minus lenses, or centre thickness with plus lenses. The relative curvature for a material is given by:

$$RC = \frac{1.523 - 1}{n_m - 1}$$

When this value is less than 1 it gives a factor by which a surface is flatter than one of the same power in crown glass of refractive index 1.523. The reduction in edge or centre thickness is indicated the factor when comparing a lens made of material *m* with one made of crown glass. The table overleaf shows a comparison of the optical properties of various plastics and glass material.

Table 16.1.

OPTICAL PROPERTIES OF WHITE PLASTICS AND GLASSES

Supplier or Manufacturer	Material	Index	V-value	Spec-Grav.	R.C.
Various	CR39	1.498	58.0	1.32	1.05
Sola	Spectralite	1.537	47.0	1.21	0.97
Signet Armorlite	RLX Lite	1.556	37.7	1.21	0.94
Younger	Youngerlite	1.556	37.7	1.21	0.94
Nikon	Nikonlite DX II	1.560	41.0	1.17	0.93
Hoya	HL-II	1.560	40.0	1.27	0.93
Essilor	Ormex	1.561	37.0	1.23	0.93
Nikon	Nikonlite II	1.580	34.5	1.47	0.90
Various	Polycarbonate	1.586	30.0	1.20	0.89
UK Optical	Alphalite 16	1.592	36.0	1.37	0.88
Primlands	TFE 160	1.594	36.7	1.34	0.88
Pentax	Superthin 1.6	1.600	36.0	1.34	0.87
Norville	Norlite 1.60	1.600	30.0	1.38	0.87
Toray	Uvithin	1.609	32.0	1.41	0.86
Various	Crown	1.523	58.9	2.54	1.00
Corning	Low Mass Crown	1.523	53.0	2.38	1.00
Pilkington	Slimline 640	1.600	41.0	2.58	0.87
Corning	Titanium 1.6	1.600	41.4	2.60	0.87
Schott	S1018	1.601	42.2	2.67	0.87
DESAG	Hi-Crown 42	1.604	41.8	2.67	0.87
Pilkington	Slimline 730	1.700	30.0	2.99	0.75
Pilkington	Slimline 750	1.700	50.8	3.38	0.75
Schott	Highlite	1.701	31.0	2.99	0.75
Schott	Tital 40	1.701	39.5	3.20	0.75
Corning	Titanium	1.701	41.5	3.16	0.75
Hoya	LHI	1.702	40.2	2.99	0.75
DESAG	Lantal	1.800	35.4	3.62	0.65
Corning	Lanthanum	1.804	35.0	3.66	0.65
Hoya	THI-II	1.806	33.3	3.47	0.65
Nikon	Pointal	1.830	32.0	3.59	0.63

Refractive Index and Lens Thickness

It should be obvious that lenses are thinner when made in a material of a higher refractive index. If demonstration lenses are cut in half and viewed from the side it presents a convincing argument to the patient. Figure 16.1 illustrates this.

Edge thickness is dependent upon both form and centre thickness, as well as the refractive index. As minus lenses tend to be flatter as the power increases, then the centre thickness and refractive index become the main factors when considering edge thickness.

$$F = \frac{n'-n}{r}$$ If n' increases and F remains constant, r also increases. If the centre thickness remains the same, [and the aperture], the increased radius of curvature must result in a decrease in edge thickness.

Fig.16.1 - sections through –10.00D lenses illustrating the reduction in edge thickness obtained with a higher refractive index.

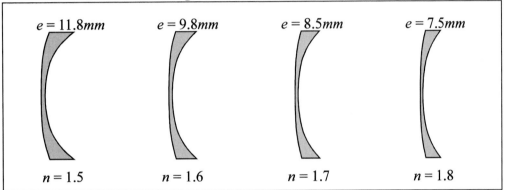

The relative curvature factor referred to previously gives an approximate idea as to the relative reduction in minus lens edge thickness compared with the same in spectacle crown glass. In order to ascertain the accuracy of this approximation, let us look at a series of minus lenses made in glasses of refractive indices 1.50, 1.60, 1.70 and 1.80. Consider the Minimum Tangential Error best form criterion for each lens, a 1.0*mm* centre thickness and a 50*mm* diameter. [Fig.16.1]. By inspection of these simple calculations shown in Table 16.1, it can be seen how accurately the relative curvature [RC] expression predicts the thickness reduction for –10.00D lenses. If the factor had predicted the edge thickness reduction precisely then the ratio in the table would have been 1.00. For the –10.00D lens it can be seen that the error is not more than 5%. It can be seen that for lower powers the RC factor over-estimates the reduction, and for higher power powers it under-estimates it. Thus, for powers over –10.00D, the actual reduction in edge thickness will be even more impressive than the RC factor would indicate.

Relative curvature is a good practical predictor of the saving in edge thickness that can be achieved in minus lenses by the use of materials of higher refractive index. The reduction is about 13% with 1.6 index, 25% with 1.7 index and 35% with 1.8 index lenses as compared with a lens of the same power in glass of refractive index 1.523.

V-value and off-axis vision

When you look through a point on a lens away from the optical centre, a prismatic effect is introduced with the base-apex line passing through the optical centre. The name given to this meridian is the *tangential meridian* and the dispersion of light due to *transverse chromatic aberration* [TCA] occurs in this meridian. This gives rise to what is referred to as *tangential blur.*[see Figure 16.2]. TCA is given by the expression:

$$TCA = \frac{P}{V}$$

where **P** is the prismatic effect at the point on the lens and **V** is the V-value. Since the prismatic effect is $P = cF$, to a very close approximation from Prentice's Rule, the

$$TCA = \frac{cF}{V},$$

from which we see the well-known fact that tangential blur is proportional to the V-value. In other words tangential blur is at its worst at the periphery of high-powered lenses, but it can be kept to a minimum by choosing a material with a high V-value.

Fig.16.2 Tangential blur when viewing through an off-axis point on a spectacle lens.

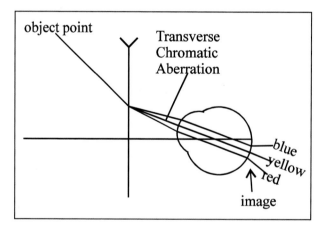

The patient complains of blur [TCA] when the object contrast is low and the retinal image is close to the resolution limit. With high contrast objects however, such as a window bar seen against a bright sky, the patient is more likely to see coloured fringes on the edges of the bar.

Density and Specific Gravity

There is often some confusion over the terms density and specific gravity. Density is defined as:

$$density = \frac{mass}{volume}$$

Specific gravity, or the density of a material relative to the density of water, is given by:

$$\frac{specific}{gravity} = \frac{density\ of\ material}{density\ of\ water}$$

If the densities are measured in grammes per cubic centimetre then the density of water is **1.00 g/cm³**, which results in the specific gravity having the same numerical value as the density of the material. It follows therefore that the units [**g/cm³**] should always be used when quoting density, whereas with specific gravity the units cancel out leaving a pure number.

Figures 16.3 and 16.4 show the calculated weights and thicknesses of a series of lenses of different powers, all made with the same diameter and edge thickness. As one would expect, lenses made in higher indices are always thinner than those made in lower values of material.

However there is a bonus in terms of weight. Glass high index materials are always denser than crown glass, but at the higher powers, due to the saving in lens volume brought about by the use of high refractive index material, the lens weight is actually less than the 'lighter' material.

So far, comparisons have been made between plus lenses of similar edge thickness and negative power lenses of the same centre thickness, but in practice this is unlikely to be the case. If we take negative power lenses, it has been conventional to have a minimum centre thickness of 1.8-2.0*mm* in CR39, and down to 0.8*mm* in some cases in glass. This centre thickness will obviously affect the edge thickness of the finished lens - it is no good having a lens material of high refractive index if the minimum lens thickness has to be considerably thicker than crown or CR39 for mechanical stability. Thus, the manufacture of high index lenses with the minimum possible centre substance has become a major aim of producers of large lenses.

In the case of plus lenses, the controlling thickness is the minimum acceptable value at the farthest point from the optical centre in the edged lens. To obtain this minimum value requires an accurate prediction of uncut diameter before surfacing, otherwise finished lenses will be produced with unacceptably thick edges.

This means that when comparing the physical data of lens materials, as shown in Table **16**.1, this is only a starting point in predicting the weight and thickness of the finished lens. You also need to know how thin lenses can safely be made for minus prescriptions, and you need a prescription manufacturer who can accurately produce plus lenses to a minimum edge thickness, if you are going to get the best result from using a high index material.

An increasing trend is to use front surface aspheric curves on single vision high index spectacle lenses to further reduce weight and thickness, by giving an optically acceptable flatter lens form.

Fig.16.3 Lens thickness comparisons for two glass and one plastics material.

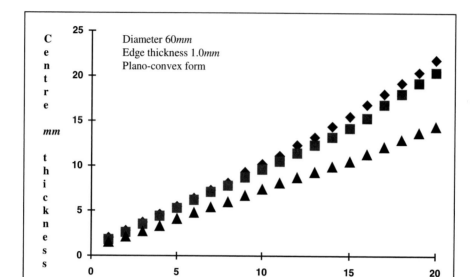

Fig.16.4 Lens weight comparison for two glass and one plastics material

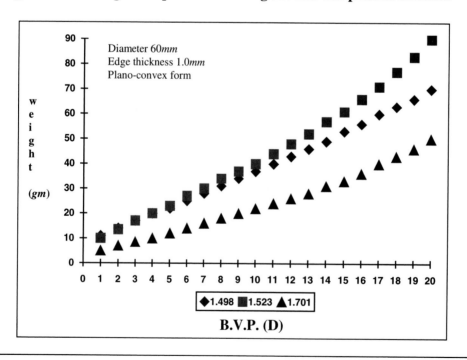

A final point which needs to be considered with the dispensing of high index materials concerns surface reflection. The amount of light reflected from a lens surface is given by:-

$$r = \left(\frac{n - n'}{n + n'}\right)^2 \times 100\%$$

where r = surface reflectivity
n = refractive index of lens material
n' = refractive index of the substance in which the lens is immersed.

From this it can be seen that as the material index increases, r will also increase. This means more surface reflection.

Using this formula and substituting the index values for the standard lens material, Table 16.2 shows the difference in surface reflections.

Light loss from CR39 and spectacle crown does not cause too many problems - except for some ghost imaging when lenses are used for night driving or at dusk. However it can be seen from the table that the higher index materials have unacceptable levels of light loss. A loss of much more than 10% is questionable and most users would find loss of more than 12-13% unacceptable.

For this reason it is recommended that any lens with an index of 1.6 or higher should have an anti-reflection coating. This is a must for lenses with indices of 1.8 and above.

Table 16.2 Losses due to reflection for a range of materials

Material	Index	Light loss*(%)	Light transmitted*(%)
CR39	1.491	7.6	92.4
Spectacle crown	1.523	8.4	91.6
Polycarbonate	1.586	10.0	90.0
Mid-index crown	1.604	10.5	89.5
Dense flint glass	1.706	13.1	86.9
Dense flint glass	1.800	15.7	84.3
Dense flint glass	1.803	16.5	83.5
Dense flint glass	1.900	18.3	81.7

* Total light loss and transmission for both surfaces.

Table 16.3 Classification by refractive index

Classification term	Refractive index [1]
Normal index	≥ 1.48 but < 1.54
Mid index	≥ 1.54 but < 1.64
High index	≥ 1.64 but < 1.74
Very High index	≥ 1.74
[1]Determined using light at a wavelength specified in BS 7017 : 1988	

17. HIGH-POWERED LENSES

General considerations

High power lenses have several inherent drawbacks from the wearer's point of view. They are thicker than 'normal', which tends to make them conspicuous if not unsightly. An increase in weight inevitably accompanies the extra thickness. On top of all this, they also alter the appearance of the wearer around the eyes, making them look unnaturally small in the case of minus lenses and large with plus lenses. There are other drawbacks with minus lenses. One becomes aware of a series of concentric images of the edge, which are known as *power rings*. These are formed by repeated reflections and appear to be situated within the lens with successive rings becoming fainter from the margin inwards. Although invisible to the wearer except in a mirror, they nevertheless draw attention from outside observers to the thick-edged lenses. Plus lenses also suffer from weight and thickness problems but this time we are concerned with centre thickness and the bulbous appearance of large lenses together with the magnifying effect they have on the wearer's eyes.

Methods of overcoming these problems need to be carefully considered, rarely in isolation, but more usually as a combination and often a compromise of solutions. The wide choice of materials, and by this I mean the ever growing variety of refractive indices in both glass and plastics, are the answer to many of the issues to be considered with high-powered lenses. These have been largely covered in the preceding chapter. Associated problems of constringence and oblique visual performance have also been dealt with in earlier chapters.

Another way of controlling the edge thickness and/or weight is by the use of *lenticulars*. Round, oval and profile lenticulars have been with us for a long time. More recently, the blended lenticular has made its appearance. Here the back surface of a high minus lens is made as a continuous surface which still has optic and margin portions, but the two are made to blend together. Several types of blended lenticular are available: Ultrablend, Wrobel Super Lenti, Lentilux, Myodisc, Omega and Aphal.

There are three cosmetic advantages of blended lenticulars. Firstly, the edge or centre thickness is much reduced, improving the appearance of the spectacles, reducing the lens weight and in the case of minus lenses, lessening the power ring reflections. In the case of Lentilux, the margin is plane, or nearly so, and has a maximum edge thickness not exceeding 5*mm*. The mean edge thickness across the power range is only 3.5*mm*.

The second advantage of blended lenticulars is that the lens appears very much like a relatively weak powered full aperture lens. Larger lenses can be dispensed. Close inspection is required to notice the change in curvature from the optic zone to the margin. The third advantage is that the magnification to the wearer's cheeks and temples is almost totally absent. Table 17.1 indicates the power ranges and available blended lenticulars.

Table 17.1 Power ranges of available blended lenticulars

Lens	Supplier	Material	Power range
Aphal	Zeiss	CR39	+5.25 to +19.00 in stronger meridian, cyl to +4.00
Lentilux	Rodenstock	1.7 glass	−6.00 to −24.00, cyl to 4.00
Myodisc	Norville	CR39	−10.00 to −25.00, cyl t0 +6.00
Omega	Essilor	CR39	+6.00 to +20.00 in stronger meridian, cyl to +6.00
Ultrablend	MW	1.7 glass	−7.25 to −17.25 plus cyl front surface, cyl to +6.00
Wrobel Super Lenticular	Norville	1.523	−5.25 to −9.75
		1.523-1.601	−10.00 to −11.75
		1.601	−12.00 to −17.00
		1.701	−17.25 to −23.00
		1.801	−23.25 to −50.00

Where higher powers are concerned it is important to discuss the form of the lenses with the supplier. A cylindrical correction is generally incorporated as a minus or plus cylinder on the front surface, rather than a back toroidal surface since the latter would present cosmetic problems in lenticular form. Even with spherical corrections, it may not be possible to produce a plane front surface in some designs with these high powers.. The result may be biconcave forms for very high minus lenses and consequently an accompanying bad oblique performance. For example, a −30.00D lens in 1.7 index glass, made with a plano front surface, has an oblique power − 30.51DS/−0.30DC for a 35° object field. Made with a −10.00 front surface the oblique power is −31.76DS/−2.57DC! This latter form in CR39 has an oblique performance of −34.68DS/−4.01DC!!

A patient who changes to blended lenticulars from the visible variety needs to be warned of some slight adaptation problems. More head movement is required because the useable area is slightly less than in some visible lenticulars, and obviously considerably less than with full aperture lenses. Many patients consider this to be a small disadvantage compared with the marked improvement in the cosmetic appearance.

Power rings formed by internal reflections from light arising from and near the edge of the minus lens are less troublesome than before anti-reflection coatings were introduced. These coatings are advisable for all distance corrections and also with near vision corrections where reflections from the lens surface may be troublesome. Some additional measures which may be used to reduce power rings even further are:

1. Edge coating
2. Edge painting
3. Tinting
4. Mini-bevel
5. Dark, thick rims for the frame
6. Blended lenticulars

All are designed to reduce the amount of light coming from the edge of the lens, and in the case of blended lenticulars, to reduce the extent of the light source, the edge itself.

Consideration of frame choice is all important for both minus and plus high powered lenses. In the case of the former, the smaller the eyesize and decentration, the better. There are various charts, tables and devices available to illustrate the edge thickness of lenses in different refractive indices and diameters. As far as high powered plus lenses are concerned we have to consider the field of view at the limit of the lens aperture. Figures 17.1 and 17.2, taken from the Essilor catalogue illustrate the annular scotoma effect and how it is much reduced with a polynomial aspheric lens.

Hence, besides removing the 'fried egg' appearance of a lenticular, the smoothly flattening polynomial curve reduces the prismatic effect at the edge of the lens and thereby makes the annular scotoma effect negligible. In a 40*mm* diameter +12.00 aspheric lenticular, as opposed to a polynomial aspheric, the deviation of a ray at 35° ocular rotation is a little less than 14°. This is the size of the annular scotoma for a fixation field of view. At 50*mm* distance from the patient that means an object 12.5*m* wide is occluded. Any lens which helps to reduce annular scotoma must, therefore, be beneficial.

Fitting the lens as close as possible to the eye increases the field of view and lessens the impact of annular scotoma. Figure 17.1(a) shows how the object **A** is occluded in the primary position of gaze, but on rotating the eye in (b) object **A** pops into view but object **B** disappears - the *Jack-in-the-box* effect. The problem is not quite as pronounced as is sometimes inferred to be in that most patients are able to move their gaze from the primary position and rarely look 35° from the primary position. Besides it is not very comfortable.

Fig.17.1 The effect of annular [ring] scotoma - Jack-in-the box effect

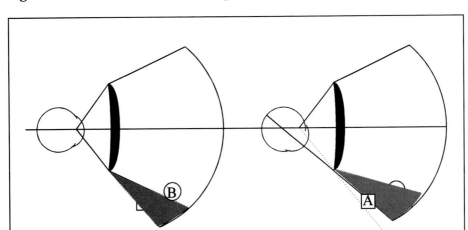

Fig.17.2 Reduced prismatic effect at the edge of the optic zone reduces ring scotoma in a polynomial aspheric.

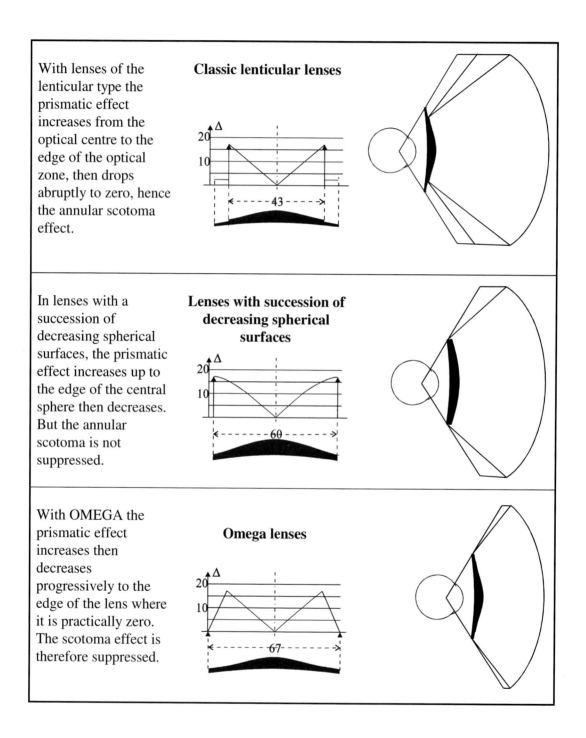

As lens power increases, previously insignificant factors affect lens function from its initial design through its final positioning before the eye. Unless compensation for these influences is made, the finished product fails to perform as anticipated.

Lens power as related to position

The principal point of focus of a lens of given power is located at a specific point. When the lens is moved, the point of focus moves as well. If a lens position must be changed but the position of the focal point must not change, a new lens power is required

For example, if a camera has a distance of +10 *cm* from the lens to the film, there is only one power of lens that will cause an object at infinity to focus on the film. The proper lens power may be calculated knowing that the focal length of the lens must be +10*cm*.

Since:

$$F = \frac{1}{f'}$$

then

$$F = \frac{1}{0.1} = +10.00D$$

If, however, the camera has a distance of +12.5*cm* from lens to film, the +10.00D lens is inappropriate, since it would focus light 2½*cm* in front of the film, producing a blurry image. This is true whether the film moves or the lens moves. As long as the distance between lens and film changes from +10 to +12.5*cm*, the power of the lens must be changed. To focus on the film at a distance of +12.5*cm*, a power of +8.00D is required - less power than for the shorter distance (Fig. 17.3).

Fig.17.3

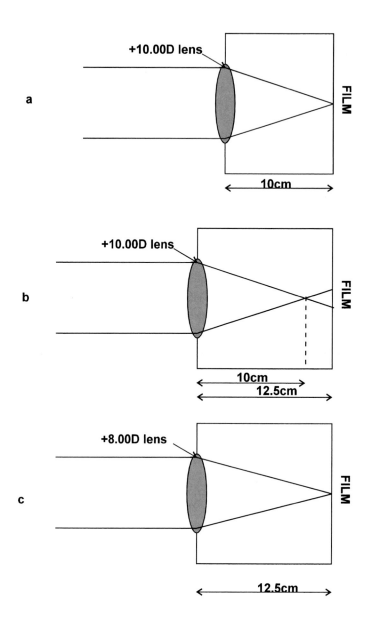

Positional lens power problems

Problem 1: If a lens of power +5.00D is mounted so as to focus light on a small screen, what new power lens will be required if the lens mounting is moved 5cm farther away from the screen?

Solution: A +5.00D lens has a focal length of +20cm. We know, then, that the mounting was originally 20cm away from the screen. If the mounting is moved 5cm farther from the screen, it is now 25cm away. To cause parallel rays of light to focus on the screen, a lens with a focal length of +25cm must be chosen. The reciprocal of 0.25m is 4. Therefore, a +4.00D lens must be chosen.

Problem 2: Parallel light enters an optical system and must be made to diverge. A −12.50D lens gives the correct amount of divergence. The system is redesigned, and this lens must be moved 2cm to the right (light is assumed to be travelling from left to right). According to the new system the light must still diverge as if from the same point. What new lens power must be used at the new location to give the same effect?

Solution: The situation described is shown in Fig.17.4. In the old system, since the focal length of a −12.50D lens is −8cm, light appeared as if it were coming from a point 8cm to the left of the lens. The new system requires that this point be maintained, but the lens must now be 2cm farther from it. The old lens may not be used, since moving it 2cm to the right would also move the focal point 2cm to the right. To maintain the integrity of the system the focal length of the new lens must be 2cm longer than that of the old, which is (8cm + 2cm or) 10cm. The diverging lens, which has a focal length of −10cm, is a −10.00D lens.

Fig.17.4

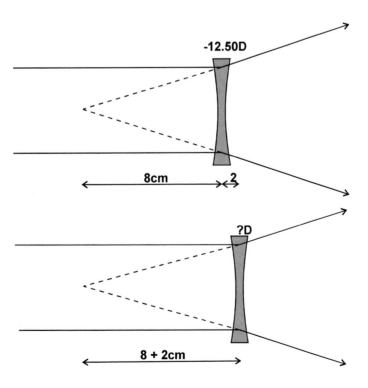

Effective power

The power of a lens is normally designated with respect to the position in space the lens occupies. It can also be designated with respect to how much vergence power it has at some point of reference. The vergence power a lens has at a position other than that position occupied by the lens itself is known as the **effective power** of the lens. The effective power of a given lens in air may be obtained by taking the reciprocal of the distance in air from the focal point of the lens to the new point of reference. (Fig.17.5)

For example, if light rays are converging towards a given point in air, when these rays are 10cm away from the point of focus they have a vergence of + 10.00D. One centimetre closer, the same rays now have a vergence of 1/0.09 or +11.11D. Still another centimetre closer and the vergence will be 1/0.08 or +12.50D.

Basically, the effective power of a lens may be thought of as being that power lens which is required to replace the original lens at a new position and yet still maintain the same focal point. If, then, a +10.00D lens is to be replaced by another lens positioned 2 cm to the right, it must be replaced by a +12.50D lens. At a position 5cm to the right, a +20.00D lens would be required. (Fig.17.6)

Fig.17.5

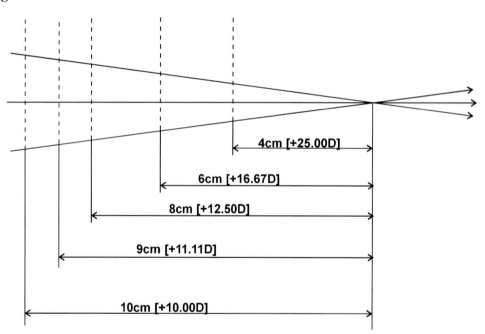

Effective power as related to vertex distance changes

The distance from the back surface of the spectacle lens to the front surface of the wearer's eye is known as the **vertex distance**. Traditionally, for purposes of calculation, a distance of 13.5mm was considered average. In actual practice, vertex distances vary considerably, ranging anywhere from 5 to 26mm and beyond. Positioning the glasses at a vertex distance other than that used during the refraction means that the effective power at the refracting distance is now different from that originally intended. For low powered lenses whose focal length is long in comparison to the vertex distance, there is very little difference. But for higher powered lenses, a small change in vertex distance can make a considerable change in effective power.

Fig.17.6

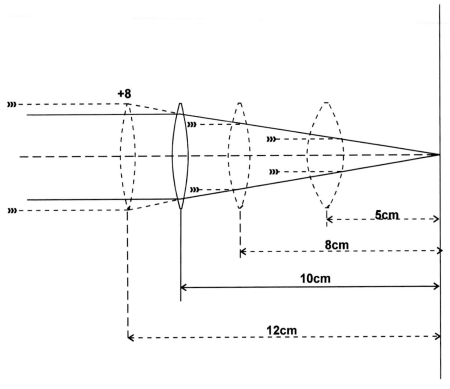

For example: A person is refracted at a 12.0*mm* vertex distance and found to need a +8.50*D* lens. A frame selection is made and the lenses fitted at a 17*mm* vertex distance. What power lens must be used at 17*mm* to give the same effective power at the refracting distance?

Solution: A +8.50*D* lens has a focal length of +11.765*cm*. If the new lens has a vertex distance of 17*mm*, this is 5*mm* to the left of the original position. To achieve the same refractive effect for the wearer, the focal length of the lens dispensed must be 5*mm* longer than for the refractive lens.

$$+11.765cm + 0.5cm = +12.265cm$$

If the new focal length must be +12.265*cm*, the new lens power must be:

$$\frac{1}{0.12265m} = +8.15D$$

Effective power of a sphero-cylinder lens

When calculating the new power needed for a sphero-cylinder lens at an altered vertex distance, the power in each major meridian must be considered separately.

For example: If a +11.00/+3.00 × 180 lens is prescribed at 12*mm* vertex distance and the frame selected is to be positioned at 15*mm*, what will the new R_x be?

Solution: The major meridians are

$$F_{180} = +11.00D$$
$$F_{90} = +14.00D$$

First F_{180} is calculated as follows:

$$f_{180} = \frac{1}{11.00} = +9.09cm$$

The new lens will be 15 minus 12, or 3*mm* farther from the line foci of the lens. Therefore since the lens is plus the focal lengths will be 3*mm* longer.

New $f_{180} = +9.09cm +0.3cms = 9.39cms$

So new $F_{180} = +10.65D$

To find the new power in the 90 degree meridian,

Since $F_{90} = +14.00D$ then $f_{90} = +7.14cms$

New $f_{90} = +7.14 +0.3 = +7.44cms$

Therefore new $F_{90} = +13.44D$

If $F_{180} = +10.65D$ and $F_{90} = +13.44D$, then the new lens power will be +10.65/+2.79 × 180. Not only has the sphere power changed, but also the power of the cylinder.   In this case it is not valid to calculate the power of the sphere (+11.00*D*), then independently the power of the cyl (+3.00*D*). The cylinder value is the difference between two meridians and not an independent entity.

As a lens becomes thicker, there is an increase in distance between front and back surfaces. Changing the position of the first lens surface with respect to the second means that the effective power of the first surface at the plane of the second surface is no longer the same. This in turn causes a change in total lens power. The actual amount is calculated using vergence.

While aphakia is something that dispensing opticians will rarely need to concern themselves with, lessons we have learned from years of dealing with aphakes have put us in good stead for dealing with the more common cases of high-powered hyperopic prescriptions. There is also the chance that you will come across the occasional aphakic patient and we need to know how to deal with their problems.

High minus lenses and negative lenticulars

As with hyperopes, myopes (particularly those with very high powers) face problems, albeit fewer than aphakes but no less significant. Myopes experience an image size smaller than that produced by the naked eye. The higher the power, the smaller the image size. This has implications for their visual acuity and leads many myopes to consider contact lenses.

A corollary to the reduced image size, though, is an improved real field of view. Indeed, unlike hyperopes and aphakes who have an area missing from their total field (the ring scotoma), myopes have an area where they will receive two images: one blurry one from behind their spectacles and one through their lenses. So a myope wearing lenticular lenses would have a comparable real field of view to a hyperope (with the same dioptric power) wearing full-field lenses.

Just as they suffer from the opposite magnification effect of hyperopes, so too do they suffer from the opposite effect to their appearance. Minus lenses make a myope's eyes appear smaller. The lenses also reveal the sides of the temples through the lenses. In very high powers this effect can be dramatic (and most undesirable).

Myopes suffer from multiple reflections from their thicker edges giving a sort of tunnel appearance. Let us consider the lens type and material options available to the myope.

Lens types
Minus lenticular

Like the plus lenticular, this lens also looks like a fried egg, but only from the front. It has a minus optical aperture surrounded by a plus 'chamfer' producing a lens of minimum edge thickness. The plus chamfer is calculated to bring the edge thickness down from the thickness of the minus power aperture at its diameter to the required edge thickness at the lens diameter, plus chamfers normally have a power of about +9.00D.

Myodisc

This lens is identical to the minus lenticular, with the exception that the chamfer is plano instead of plus. Thus, the edge thickness of the finished lens is the same as that of the minus power aperture.

Blended lenticular

In the blended lenticular the optical aperture is blended into the flange, eliminating the obvious line and improving the appearance. The spectacles will also be much lighter and more comfortable, given the reduction in thickness of the lenses. The final weight will obviously depend on the material chosen. While aphakes and high plus lens wearers are generally restricted to CR-39 or high-index plastics, myopes do have the option of high-index glass, limited only by the material available. These were discussed in the last chapter.

Fig.17.7. Minus lenticular lens

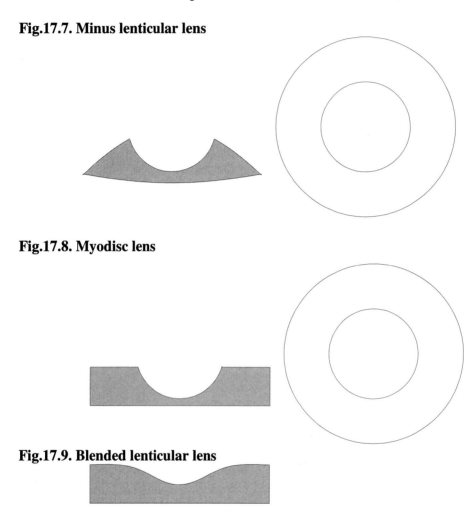

Fig.17.8. Myodisc lens

Fig.17.9. Blended lenticular lens

Vergence of light as it travels through a lens

When light strikes a lens, it is refracted at the front surface, then travels through the thickness of the lens. It is again refracted when reaching the back lens surface. For thin lenses, the distance travelled from front to back surfaces makes no appreciable change in total lens power. The thicker the lens becomes, however, the more of a discrepancy there is between nominal power ($F_1 + F_2$) and the actual measured power of the lens. As light strikes F_1 its vergence is changed. It is caused to converge or diverge to a greater or lesser extent than previously. It has an additional vergence change when reaching F_2. For a thin lens, when the vergence of the entering light is zero (parallel rays) the light exiting the lens has a vergence equal to $F_1 + F_2$. For example, if $F_1 = +5.00D$ and $F_2 = +1.00D$, when light strikes F_1 it is caused to converge. It now has a vergence of $+5.00D$. Because the lens is thin, it immediately strikes the back surface before its vergence changes and is caused to converge an additional dioptre, so on leaving F_2 it has a vergence of $+6.00D$. For a thick lens the converging light would have a chance to travel a given distance before reaching F_2. As will be recalled from the previous section on effective power, as this converging or diverging light continues to travel through the lens, by the time it reaches the second surface, F_2, it will have a slightly different vergence from when it left F_1. This is because it is now a different distance from its plane of reference. It is this new vergence (the effective power of F_1 at F_2) that F_2 alters to produce an exiting vergence.

Vergence of light striking F_2

For a thick lens, after light has left the first surface, F_1, it travels for a time in glass, having a refractive index higher than that of air. Because vergence depends on the relationship between refractive index and distance ($L = n/\ell$), the vergence of light leaving F_1 and striking F_2 may not be calculated in terms of distance alone.

Initially one would think that the new vergence would be found by directly adding or subtracting lens thickness from the image distance of light leaving the first surface (ℓ'). This was the case in previous effective power problems, and in air this proves true. Instead, however, it is necessary to find the new vergence by adding or subtracting the reduced thickness of the lens from the reciprocal of the vergence. This keeps the reference medium as air, which is the better choice since calculations are easier when the final results are for rays converging or diverging in air.

For Example: Parallel light enters a $7mm$ thick lens that has a front surface power of $+12.00D$ and a refractive index of 1.523. What vergence will the light have when striking F_2? Solution: After leaving F_1, the light has a vergence that can be calculated as follows:

Substituting the correct numerical values, we find:

$$+12.00D = L_1' - 0$$
$$\text{or } L_1' = +12.00D$$

Light leaving F_1 has a vergence of $+12.00D$. The light is now converging toward a point to the right of F_1. That point in air would be found by taking the reciprocal of the vergence.

$$L_1' = \frac{1}{\ell_1'} \quad \text{and}$$

$$+12.00 = \frac{1}{\ell_1'}$$

$$\ell_1' = +0.0833m$$

The distance in question $+0.0833m$.

However, the light must travel through glass for *7mm* before reaching air. To find the vergence of light at F_2, the *reduced thickness* of this lens must be subtracted from $\ell_1{'}$ because the point of focus is now closer to the new plane of reference, which is the back surface of the lens. Therefore the new distance (ℓ_2) is:

$$\ell_2 = \ell_1{'} - \frac{t}{n}$$

where $\frac{t}{n}$ is the reduced thickness of the lens.

(Thickness must be expressed in the same units as $\ell_1{'}$).

$$\ell_2 = 0.0833 - \frac{0.007}{1.523} m$$
$$= 0.0833 - 0.0046 = 0.0787m$$

The vergence of the light entering F_2 is the reciprocal of $0.0787m$.

$$L_2 = \frac{1}{\ell_2}$$
$$= \frac{1}{0.0787}$$
$$= +12.71D$$

The vergence of light entering F_2 is $+12.71D$. It can be seen from the above example that if F_2 were plano, then the vergence of light leaving F_2 would also be $+12.71D$. This is not the result that would be expected if lens power were assumed to be the sum of the two lens surface powers.

Front and back vertex powers

It has been shown that because of lens thickness the nominal power of a lens does not always equal the actual power of the lens. It will be recalled that when parallel light enters the front of a lens, it is refracted and exit from the rear surface of the lens. The image, be it real or virtual, falls at the second principal focus.

The reciprocal of the distance in air from the rear surface of the lens to the second principal focus is a specific measure of the power of this lens and is known as the ***back vertex power*** ($F_v{'}$). (This is the measure of power of most importance in ophthalmic lenses).

Also, in review, if parallel light enters from the rear surface? the place where the image now forms is known as the first principal focus. The reciprocal of the distance in air from the front surface to the first principal focus is another measure of the power of the lens and is referred to as the *front vertex power* (F_v) (Fig.17.10). It is not unusual to find front and back vertex powers to be different. If the lens is equi-concave or equiconvex, the front and back vertex powers will be the same. If the lens has any other form and is thick, there may be a measurable difference between the two.

Calculating front and back vertex powers

Front and back vertex powers may be found by finding vergences as light approaches and leaves each lens surface. They may also be found using a formula summarising the necessary vergence factors. Following the vergence methods as introduced earlier for solving this type of problem will give a much better understanding of the action of a lens upon light than will simple formula memorisation. Both methods are presented.

Fig.17.10

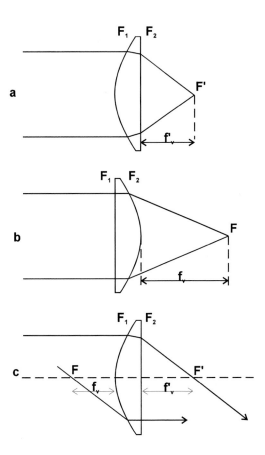

If light enters a lens as parallel rays, the back vertex power of a lens will be equal to the vergence these light rays have when leaving the lens. If the form, thickness, and refractive index of that lens are known, the back vertex power may be found by systematically tracing the path light rays take through the lens.

For Example: If a lens has dimensions of $F_1 = +8.00D$, $F_2 = -2.00D$, $t = 5mm$ and $n = 1.523$, what is the back vertex power of the lens?

Solution: Light entering the lens must be from an object at infinity to accurately determine back vertex lens power. The rays entering the front surface of the lens will then be parallel, having a vergence of zero (Fig.17.11).

Since $L_1{'} = F_1 + L_1$

and $L_1 = 0.00D$
then $L_1' = +8.00D + 0.00D$
or $L_1' = +8.00D$

To find the vergence of light at F_2, the reduced thickness is subtracted from ℓ_1'.

$$\ell_2 = \ell_1' - \frac{t}{n}$$
$$= \frac{1}{8.00} - \frac{0.005}{1.523}m$$
$$= 0.125 - 0.0033$$
$$= 0.1217m$$

Therefore the vergence of light at F_2 is
$$L_1 = \frac{1}{\ell_1} = \frac{1}{0.1217} = +8.22D$$

(This is the same procedure as finding the effective power of F_1 at F_2.)

Now since $L_2' = F_2 + L_2$
then in this case $L_2' = -2.00 + 8.22$
$$= +6.22$$

Since back vertex power is the vergence with which light from an object at infinity leaves a lens, the back vertex power (F_v') for this lens is +6.22D and the principal focus is +16.07cm behind the lens. This is noticeably different from the nominal power of the lens, which comes out equal to +6.00D with its principal focus +16.67cm behind the lens.

Fig.17.11

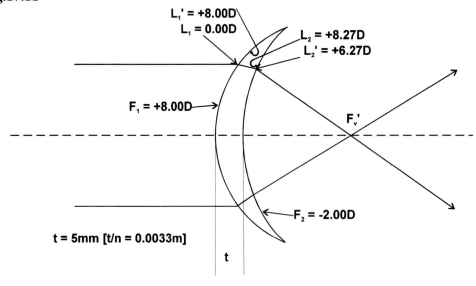

Problem: What would the front vertex power be for the lens described in the previous problem?

Solution: To simplify the construction, it is easier to find F_v, the front vertex power, by turning the lens around and considering light to be entering from the back (Fig.17.10). In this manner, then, sign conventions are maintained and less confusion results. The same methodology may be used as in finding the back vertex power. To avoid confusion in terminology the back surface of the lens now becomes F_1 (since light now enters it as if it were the front surface), and the front surface will become F_2 (Fig.17.12).

$$\text{and } L_1 = 0.00D$$
$$\text{with the new } F_1 = -2.00D$$
$$\text{then } L_1' = -2.00D + 0.00D$$
$$= -2.00D$$

Again the vergence of light at F_2 is found as reduced thickness subtracted from l_1'

$$\ell_2 = \ell_1' - \frac{t}{n}$$
$$= \frac{1}{-2.00} - \frac{0.005}{1.523}m$$
$$= -0.50 - 0.0033$$
$$= -0.05033m$$

$$L_1 = \frac{1}{\ell_1} = \frac{1}{-0.05033} = -1.99D$$

Now $L_1' = F_1 + L_1$

$$L_1' = +8.00 - 1.99D$$
$$= +6.01D$$

The front vertex power for this lens is $+6.01D$, which is extremely close to the nominal power of the lens. If the surface the lens light were entering had been plano, this vertex power would have been equal to the nominal power. The more curved the entering surface, the more the vertex power of the lens will differ from its nominal power.

The previous vergence methods may be summarised into formulas. The formula for back vertex power is

$$F_v' = \frac{F_1}{1 - \frac{t}{n}F_1} + F_2$$

And that for front vertex power is

$$F_v = \frac{F_2}{1 - \frac{t}{n}F_1} + F_1$$

The above formulas give results that are accurate and identical to those found by the vergence method. Alternate formulas for front and back vertex powers derived from the above formulas using higher mathematics are

$$F_v' = F_1 + F_2 + \tfrac{t}{n}\left(F_1\right)^2$$

$$F_v = F_1 + F_2 + \tfrac{t}{n}\left(F_2\right)^2$$

Fig.17.12

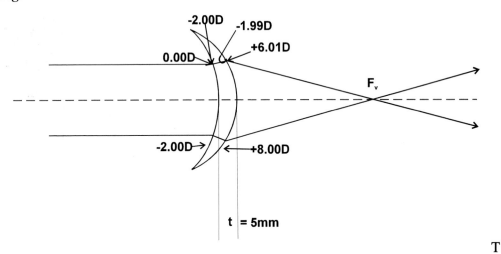

T

These formulas are approximations and, although somewhat easier to work, are not expected to give the accuracy of the more exact forms. The approximations were more widely used before small calculators became available.

The vergence error is due to the effectivity difference between the dispensed lens and the trial lens. This occurs because the trial lens has a plano front surface and the dispensed lens a high plus powered one, and because of the thickness difference.

With high powered plus lenses one of the most important facts we have to consider is the *Near Vision Effectivity Error* [NVEE]. Consider the following example where the distance Rx is +12.00D and the near vision spectacles have back vertex power +15.00D [Fig.17.14]. Assuming a plano-convex trial lens with the spherical surface towards the eye, then the reading lens will have a +15.00D back surface power. The vergence leaving the lens must be +12.00D for a clear retinal image, so taking the trial lens to be 4mm thick, calculation shows the object will be 33.1cm from the front surface of the lens.

The difference in thicknesses between the trial lens and the final dispensed lens is ignored only as far as placing the object is concerned; i.e. the object was

33.1 + 0.4 + 1.0 = 34.5cm

from the eye with the trial lens. It will be at a slightly different distance from the eye with the dispensed lens when the same distance 33.1cm is taken for the object distance from the front surface of the lens. Calculation shows that taking this slight difference into account alters the figures below by less than $0.1D$.

Firstly, manufacturers usually design their lenses for distance vision, so we take the best form for this power which is judged to be one with a back surface power of − $2.00D$ and *p*-value 0.65 for an aspheric. In the UK it is likely that the lens will be glazed with its optical centre on the horizontal centre line, some 5 or 6*mm* below the centre of the pupil in the primary position of gaze, so the lens must have a pantoscopic tilt to make its optical axis pass through the eye's centre of rotation. This a necessary lens design criterion.

Fig.17.13 Near vision correction with a 4*mm* thick plano-convex trial lens

THE SOURCE OF NEAR VISION EFFECTIVITY ERROR

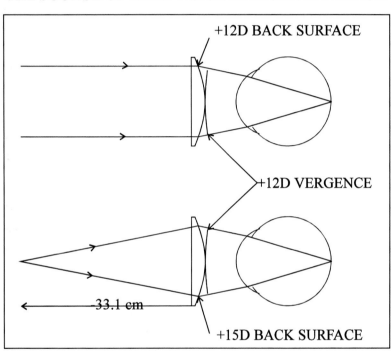

The above is a paraxial calculation, which is reasonable to assume since the trial frame will be lowered so that the patient looks through the optical centres when determining the addition and care will be taken to keep the same vertex distance. However, what happens if we order a +15.00*D* lens for near vision?

Due to near vision effectivity, the lens will be underpowered even along the axis. If the +15.00*D* lens indicated by the trial lens refraction is ordered, this means the patient is compelled to hold the object further away in order to achieve a mean oblique image vergence of +12.00*D*. The problem is usually overcome by adding a small amount of plus power to the trial lens refraction. Table 17.2 shows the amounts which should be added to the prescription for the near vision lens. By adding these amounts the patient is able to see the near work at an acceptable distance. In actual practice few people experience problems if the near vision effectivity error is not compensated for in this way.

Table 17.2 Near vision effectivity compensation

Trial lens prescription for near	Correction value for the stated Add		
	Add 2.00	**Add 2.50**	**Add 3.00**
+8.00			
+8.50			
+9.00			
+9.50			+0.25
+10.00		+0.25	
+10.50			
+11.00	+0.25		
+11.50			
+12.00			
+12.50			+0.50
+13.00			
+13.50		+0.50	
+14.00			
+14.50			
+15.00	+0.50		
+15.50			+0.75
+16.00			

To summarise the following should be carefully considered when dispensing high powered lenses:

Frames should:
- be lightweight to avoid rims adding unnecessarily to any ring scotoma
- possess adjustable pads, if possible to allow some vertical movement of the OCs to correspond with the pantoscopic tilt and allow minimum vertex distance fitting
- where possible should have a boxed centre distance as close to the patient's PD since this centres the lenses better in the frame. Excessively upswept shapes should be avoided since shaping may cut into the thicker optic zone.

The vertex distance should be kept as small as possible since that:
- maximises the field of view
- reduces convergence demand
- reduces retinal image size
- reduces the magnified appearance of the subject's eye
- reduces distortion and chromatic aberration compared with longer vertex distances.

Centration
- For single vision distance lenses, the semi-PDs should be recorded and the lenses centred accordingly, even in the case of a unilateral aphakic. Accurate centring is necessary not only to prevent differential prismatic effects but to centre the vertex of an aspherical surface. Accurate centration ensures the best oblique gaze performance with both aspheric and spherical lenses.
- Near vision lenses should be centred according to semi-NCDs.

- Bifocal segments must be inset according to the requirements to make the right and left reading portion fields of view coincide.
- Vertical centration and pantoscopic tilt must correspond.

Near vision effectivity error should be compensated.

An ultraviolet absorbing coating should be considered.

18. TINTED & PROTECTIVE LENSES

It is common sense that good sight means increased efficiency and a safer environment both at work and at play. This is an attempt to look at the hazards which can adversely effect the most valued of our senses and ways in which those hazards can be counteracted.

Health and Safety at Work regulations have sought to encourage those engaged in occupations which present potential dangers to the eyes to wear suitable protective visors or goggles, but chances are still taken particularly when it comes to radiation hazards. On any sunny day in this country, and sometimes on not so sunny days, droves of people can be seen sporting the latest trend in sunspectacles, but figures for eye accidents suggest that nearly 75% of the victims were supplied with protection but did not use it. Unfortunately employees cannot be forced to wear the protection provided.

In the past the emphasis was on mechanical injury. Although the eyes have a degree of natural protection, they are still extremely vulnerable. Below is a list of processes based on British factory legislation and for which protection is required by law.

By and large employees recognise immediate threats to their eyes from these sources. It is the hidden wavelengths of radiation which pose perhaps the greatest threat to vision. Light is that part of the spectrum of electromagnetic radiation which is perceivable to the eye [Fig.18.1]. This visible spectrum has a waveband of $\lambda = 380$ to 780 *nm* in air [**1 nanometre = $10^{-9} m$**].

Present day industrial practice seems to encourage more light on the task to increase light levels, especially for the partially sighted. Modern light sources with their high outputs and lower costs have helped to promote such attitudes. Now, however, the tables are reversed as evidence is suggesting that several diseases associated with ageing [*cataracts and retinal changes such as age-related macular degeneration in particular*], could be accelerated by excessive light, whether natural or artificial.

The blue hazards, whereby visible light at the blue end of the spectrum can be dangerous at high intensities, have only recently been recognised, and the use of darkened glasses could well be encouraged where exposures are excessive.

The precise exposure conditions, wavelengths and intensities required to injure the delicate eye tissues have not always been well understood. The hazardous levels depend considerably on age. Excessive light exposure in elderly people is particularly to be avoided, because the biological repair mechanisms at the cellular level are generally considered to become less effective with age.

Table 18.1 Eye risk processes based upon Schedule 1 of the Protection of Eyes Regulations 1974, SI 1974 No 1681.

Particles or fluids under pressure	Compressed-air shot blasting, or erosion of concrete or cleaning of buildings or structures. Cleaning by high pressure water jets. Pressure injection of liquids into buildings or structures. Compressed-air removal of swarf, dust, or dirt.
Use of power or hand tools	Striking of masonry nails by hand or power tools. Work with cartridge operated tools. Chipping of metal, removal of rivets, bolts etc. From any structure or plant by hand or power tools. Removal of surface coatings by hand or power tools [e.g. *paint, scale, rust etc.*] Using power driven high speed metal cutting saws or cutting off wheels. Driving bolts, pins, collars, etc. Into any structure or plant by hand or power tools. Metal breaking by hand or power tools. Work with a hand or power tool on glass, hard plastics, concrete, stone, brickwork etc. Fettling of metal castings including hot fettling of steel castings by flux-injected burner. Dry grinding of metals and dressing abrasive wheels. Machining of metals.
Work with molten metal, molten salts and other hot materials	Pouring or skimming molten metal in foundries. Working at molten salt baths. Work at a molten metal furnace. Foundry work where hot sand is thrown off. Work in glass manufacture. Manufacture of forgings. Pressure die-casting.
Work involving chemicals	Working at plant which contains [*or has contained*] injurious chemicals. Working at open vessels containing injurious chemicals.
Work with wire and wire cutting	Work in wire and wire rope making [*including coiling*] Cutting wire or metal strapping under tension.
Work with electric arcs, arc plasma, welding and lasers	Work involving use of an exposed electric arc or stream of arc plasma. Gas and electric arc welding. Cutting, boring, cleaning, spraying by using an apparatus to which air, oxygen or flammable gas is supplied under pressure. Work with lasers.

Fig.18.1 The Electromagnetic Spectrum

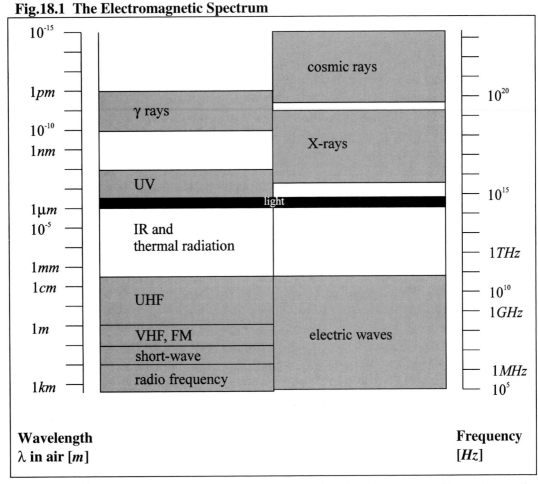

Ultraviolet radiation has long been associated with cataract formation and chronic irritation to the cornea - even keratitis often noted as sun or snow blindness. The eye's crystalline lens protects the retina, but special protection is needed by those with intra-ocular lens implants, and more and more UV absorbing IOLs are now being implanted to avoid the photochemical retinal damage which would otherwise result.

Domestic sources of UV radiation come from fluorescent and mercury discharge tubes. These are now used so widely and it is recognised that there is some benefit in screening fluorescent sources in the home with acrylic diffusers which absorb the UV component, thus protecting the eyes from damage.

The retina is eight hundred times more susceptible to ultraviolet radiation than near infra-red waves known for their heating powers. Generally two types of UV radiation are distinguished, UVB [280-320 nm] is absorbed by the cornea and UVA [320-400 nm], which is transmitted by the crystalline lens of children and the aphakic, but which is generally attenuated by the lens of an average adult. UVA makes up 97% of the total UV from the sun and produces the characteristic photokeratitis seen in snow blindness with considerable damage to the corneal epithelium, delayed some hours after exposure. The cornea absorbs all of 280 nm UVB incident upon it, but this falls to just a third when the wavelength moves into the 360 nm range [UVA]. Fortunately the anterior ocular media protect the retina from damage and less than 1% total of all UV radiation incident on the eye reaches the retina. This is, however, at the expense of the cornea, with the risk of keratitis, and to the lens with the risk of cataract.

At work, welders are most at risk from UV damage to eyes. Better known as 'arc-eye', this condition is often seen in its milder forms. The symptoms appear some 6 to 12 hours after exposure to intense sources of light of short duration and the onset of the reaction is marked by the sensation of having grit under the eyelids, accompanied by pain. Redness of the eyes and sensitivity to light are also present.

Although eye protection designed to cut out ultra-violet light reduces the radiation to a safe level, no practical solution seems to have been found to reduce the glare produced by the welding process which is troublesome to vision. The contrast between the bright emission of the welding arc and the low levels of illumination in the background, together with the small size of the arc makes the job of the welder particularly difficult and the task almost impossible to see.

Furthermore, during arc ignition normal welding goggles cause considerable problems as it is impossible to see through them before the arc has been struck. It is hardly surprising therefore, that workers are tempted to remove their eye protection just when they are most at risk.

The thermal hazard from infra-red wavelengths has been known for more than two centuries, 'glass-blowers cataract' being a typical example. Today, steel and furnace workers, locksmiths and chain makers are most at risk and should be warned of the cumulative damage which can result over a period of years.

Lasers are finding ever increasing application in such diverse fields as entertainment, supermarkets, manufacturing industry, defence and of course ophthalmology.

As powerful industrial lasers can cut several millimetres of steel as if it were tissue paper, laser light is one form of radiation which can certainly be felt. What, then are the consequences for the eyes and what should we use to protect them from laser light?

Until now, the only relevant legislation [*the 1974 Protection of Eyes Regulations*] simply makes reference to the use of 'suitable' eye protection. Even BS4803 Radiation Safety of Laser Products merely identifies some basic considerations which should be used when specifying eye protection.

In the UK, no attempt has been made so far to ensure that laser safety glasses are capable of withstanding the enormous heating effects of a laser beam. Laser users have traditionally only been able to assess the suitability of the available glasses on the basis of the quoted optical density of the material at a particular laser wavelength.

Light absorbing spectacle lenses are divided according to their degree of absorption for visible light into sun protection lenses with a transmittance of less than 80% and filter lenses with a transmittance of more than 80% [low attenuation of light]. In the UV range [with some lenses in the IR range] most of these lenses absorb more strongly than clear lenses, but no limiting values have been fixed. Examples of spectral transmissions are given in Figs. 18.2 to 18.4.

Fig.18.2 Spectral transmission curves for Zeiss filter lenses

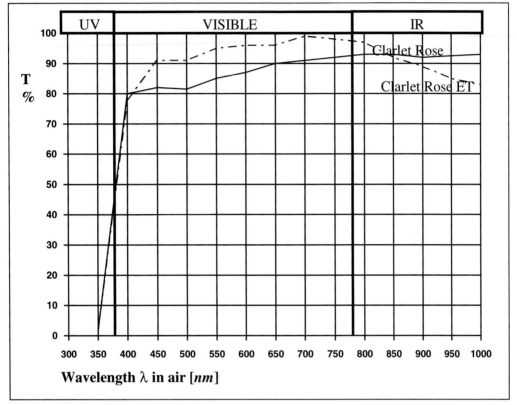

Sun protection lenses are worn to protect the eyes against glare on the one hand, and to improve visual acuity on the other. Protection is provided against the following:

- glare caused by visible light, leading to a reduction in visual acuity
- red vision [erythropsia] caused by visible, mostly green light and
- inflammation of the conjunctiva [conjunctivitis, ice or snow blindness] caused by short-wave UV radiation below $\lambda = 313$ *nm*.

In modern sunglasses attenuation of the various colours of visible light has been selected in such a way that natural colour rendition is guaranteed. Although sunglasses are useful in sunshine, their use is not advisable in twilight conditions or at night.

Filter lenses are used to avoid or reduce eyestrain and to increase visual performances by enhanced contrast. No exact explanation for this phenomenon is given. It is attributed mainly to the absorption of the longer-wave UV and blue-violet light [reduction of the scattered light or fluorescence of the crystalline lens, enhancement of image contrast].

Fig.18.3 **Spectral transmission curves for Zeiss spectacle lenses with filter anti-reflection coating [a-Clarlet ET, b-Punktal ET]**

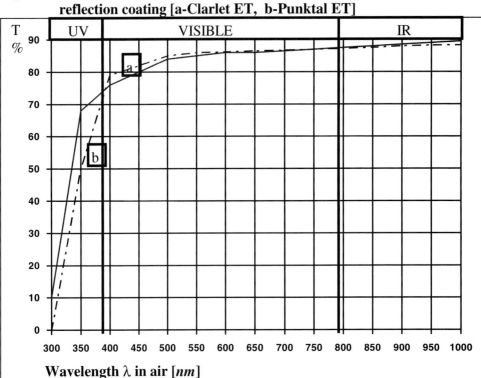

Wavelength λ in air [*nm*]

Fig.18.4 **Spectral transmission curves for Zeiss sun protection lenses a-Clarlet brown 50%, b-Umbra Punktal 65, c-Umbral 85**

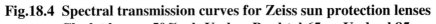
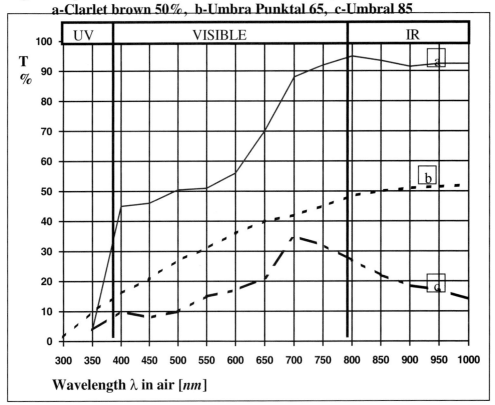

Wavelength λ in air [*nm*]

Sun protection lenses can be incorporated with any type of corrective lens. The following possibilities exist:

- Solid tinted lenses, in which the light attenuation is, however dependent upon the thickness. They are therefore mostly used as plano lenses and as fused equitint shells on clear base lenses.
- Lenses with an absorptive layer which is vacuum deposited onto the main lens. These lenses offer uniform attenuation over the whole surface, even in lenses with very high powers. The vacuum deposited coatings are as hard as glass and do not increase the weight of the lens.

For spectacle lenses made of CR39, absorptive surface coatings are generally produced by using a dipping or immersion procedure suitable for all lens powers. Standard sun protection lenses are produced with a light attenuation of up to 85%. Lenses with still higher reduction of light are protective lenses for special applications. The transmittance values for the various wavelengths for non prescription sunglasses are laid down in BS 2724[1987] Sunglare Eye Protection for General Use.

Photochromic lenses darken when exposed to short-wave radiations between about 300 nm and 450 nm. The lenses clear again when the radiation is removed. The clearing process occurs due to heat [thermal bleaching] and long-wave radiation [optical bleaching] The hue ranges from brownish-grey to bluish-grey depending on the type of glass, the temperature and the adsorptance attained. Fig.18.5 shows spectral transmission curves for a photochromic lens.

Fig.18.5 Spectral transmission curves of a photochromic borosilicate lens [thickness 2.0mm] a-unexposed, b-after exposure of 15 mins.

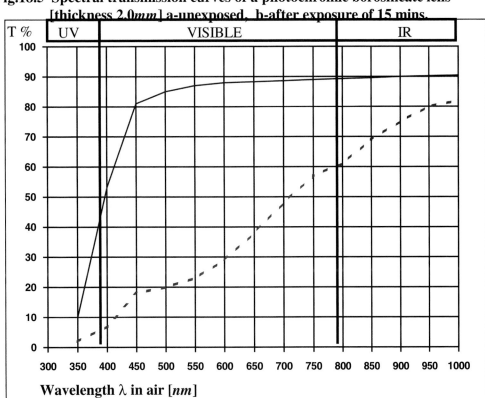

After an exposure period of 10 to 15 minutes a state of equilibrium is reached between darkening and clearing. The light transmission the present at 555 *nm* [maximum of the spectral photopic sensitivity of the eye] is known as the saturation transmission; it is dependent to a large extent on temperature.

In the 1980's, American Optical, followed by Rodenstock and Transitions, responded to the requirement for lighter weight lenses by developing photochromic plastics materials.. Glass photochromic lenses have become less temperature dependent and the fading or clearing rates in particular appear to have improved considerably, allowing lenses with a much greater change in transmittance to be used for general purposes. Table 18.2 lists materials which are currently available for prescription lenses and the transmittance ranges are given. It should be remembered that glass photochromic lenses, being solid tints, will show a variation in transmittance for given thicknesses.

Table 18.2 Prescription photochromic material transmittance ranges

Supplier	Material	100%	Luminous transmittance range	0%
Corning	Photogray Extra		88% ▬▬▬▬▬▬ 22%	
	Photobrown Ext		88% ▬▬▬▬▬▬ 22%	
Pilkington Reactolite Rapide	Borosilicate grey		91% ▬▬▬▬▬▬▬ 17%	
	Borosilicate B		90% ▬▬▬▬▬▬▬ 17%	
	Sprint brown		80% ▬▬▬▬▬▬▬	
	Sprint grey		8% ▬▬▬▬▬▬▬	
			89%	
			8%	
Zeiss	Umbramatic SR		85% ▬▬▬▬▬ 25%	
	Umbramatic SL Uromatic		85% ▬▬▬▬▬ 25%	
	Umbramatic equitint		90% ▬▬▬ 50%	
	Clarlet um/tic Tital		90% ▬▬▬▬▬ 30%	
	umbramatic		90% ▬▬▬▬▬ 30%	
			90% ▬▬▬▬▬ 30%	
Rodenstock	Colormatic 2		90% ▬▬▬ 50%	
	Colormatic SB		85% ▬▬▬▬▬ 25%	
	Colormatic 1.6		88% ▬▬▬▬ 33%	
	Perfalit colormatic		80% ▬▬▬ 35%	
Hoya	Sungray extra		88% ▬▬▬▬▬▬ 22%	
	Sunbrown extra		88% ▬▬▬▬▬▬ 22%	
	Suncity brown		90% ▬▬▬ 50%	
	Sunbrown extra2		90% ▬▬▬▬ 33%	
Norville	Photal		87% ▬▬▬▬ 42%	
	Polarised photochromic		35% ▬▬▬ 15%	
Essilor	Transition plus		82% ▬▬▬▬ 42%	
Signet	Kodak photoplastic		82% ▬▬▬▬ 42%	

A number of different reflections may occur in spectacle lenses. The various types are represented schematically in Fig.18.6. These reflections are reduced by anti-reflection coatings.

Fig.18.6 Reflections in a spectacle lens

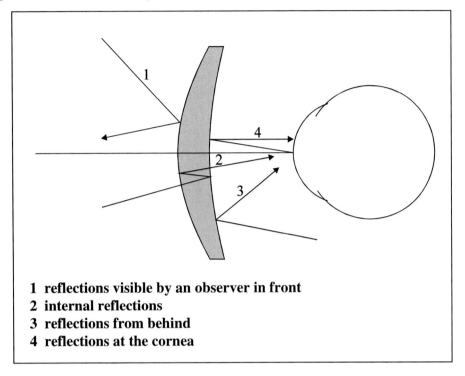

1 **reflections visible by an observer in front**
2 **internal reflections**
3 **reflections from behind**
4 **reflections at the cornea**

Although the reduction of reflections also involves an increase in transmission, this does not mean that the use of anti-reflection coatings for absorptive lenses is a contradiction in terms; their primary task is to reduce disturbing light in the finished spectacle lenses. They may indeed be particularly beneficial for light attenuating lenses which, although they reduce transmission, do not decrease the reflections on the back surface of the lenses. The spectral distribution of the transmitted light is virtually unaffected by the anti-reflection coating.

The requirements to be met by filters and equipment for personal eye-protection against laser radiation are stipulated in the West German Standard DIN 58215 and BS EN 207:1994 for the spectral range 180nm to 1000 nm on the basis of maximum permissible corneal irradiance. The permissible radiation is dependent on the wavelength and exposure time. As stated previously the eye is particularly endangered by laser radiation with wavelengths between 400 nm and 1400 nm, as the radiation in this range can be absorbed by the cornea and crystalline lens; in the radiation range between 1400 nm and 1000 μm the anterior ocular media and the area surrounding the eye may suffer damage.

Fig.18.7 Spectral transmission curve for Zeiss laser safety filter for Nd-YAG lasers

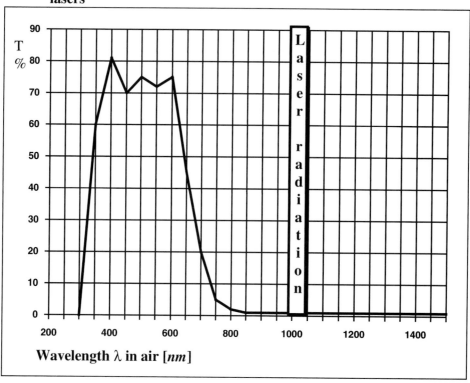

Fig.18.8 Spectral transmission curve for Zeiss laser safety filter for CO₂ lasers

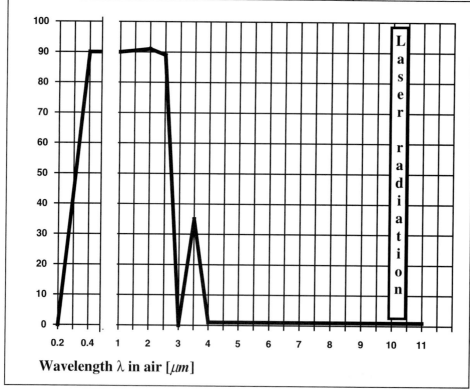

Safety filters which protect against all types of laser radiation at the same time do not exist. Laser safety filters must be suitable for the wavelength and energy of the laser used. Figs. 18.7 and 18.8 provide transmission curves for two types of laser safety filters.

As far as protection against mechanical hazards are concerned, then plastics lenses in the form of CR39 and polycarbonate are available in prescription form as well as plano form and shields. With glass which is notoriously brittle and shatters into sharp pieces when broken there are a few ways in which it can be strengthened to provide limited protection against such dangers. It can be done by making spectacle lenses in a laminated construction or by strengthening ordinary glass lenses by heat or chemical treatment.

Laminated lenses consist of a thin parallel film of a plastics material, usually polyvinyl butyral, sandwiched between two layers of annealed glass [Fig.18.9]. The three layers are firmly bonded together, the contact surfaces of each of the glass components have been accurately ground and polished to ensure good adhesion. Special care must be taken during the cementing process to exclude foreign particles of dust and dirt which embed themselves into the relatively soft plastics layer producing noticeable pits within the blank.

Fig.18.9 Laminated lens blank

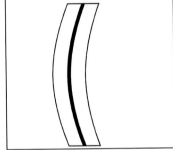

If a finished glass lens is raised to a temperature of about 650-700°C and then is rapidly cooled, it is rendered capable of withstanding the impact of quite severe blows. A lens treated in this way is termed thermally toughened. As with all safety lenses they are expected to resist breakage by surviving an impact test specified by British Standards which is updated regularly. The effect of thermally toughening is to set up a high degree of internal stress in the lens. This reveals itself as a prominent strain pattern which appears when a treated lens is placed in a strain viewer. Fig.18.10 illustrates typical strain patterns in positive and negative lenses.

Fig.18.10 Strain patterns in toughened lenses

Plus lens   **Minus lens**

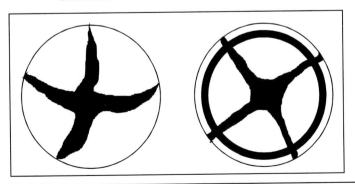

A comparable if not greater degree of impact resistance can be given to a lens by the chemical tempering process developed by Corning. The pre-heated lens is immersed for 16 hours in a bath containing molten potassium nitrate at a temperature of around 460°C. During this period there is an interchange between the potassium ions in the liquid and the sodium ions near the surface of the lens. Since the potassium ions are larger than the sodium ions which they replace there is a gradual build up of compression in a surface layer of the glass, similar to that produced by thermal toughening. Ordinary crown glass is unsuitable for this treatment.

19. LENS SURFACING/GLAZING

Mass producers of lenses make semi-finished blanks in a reasonably comprehensive range of curves and are thus able to achieve production runs at a unit cost not normally possible in 'one off' systems. Another advantage of using them is that faster delivery times of finished lenses can be realised.

As stated at the beginning of this book it was traditional at one time for opticians in the UK to have a small supply of worked uncut lenses in a limited range of prescriptions and to cut edge and fit them to stock frames on the premises. As the range of different types of lenses as well as frames increased many resorted to the use of large prescription laboratories for the supply of finished lenses if not to the supply of complete spectacles.

Both the methods of surfacing and edging lenses have made great technological advances over the years, making it easier, even if costlier, to prepare lenses for the finished product. Economic factors, and even more so, marketing strategies have seen a full circle of events whereby the surfacing and glazing of complex lenses on the premises is again commonplace. No doubt the circle will continue its cycle.

Although the production techniques are similar for glass and plastics, there are some important differences to be noted. The two materials will therefore be discussed separately, beginning with glass.

Lenses must be correctly located for the different surfacing stages and this can be done either by marking key points on the lens with a suitable ink or by jigging at the blocking stage. If jigging, whereby the lens is engraved, notched or grooved in some way, is not being used then the ink marking method must be used. The markings required on the lens vary according to the blocking system employed. In general, they must indicate the optical centre position and, when applicable, the cylinder axis and base-apex direction.

In order to hold the lens firmly and accurately for surfacing, a metal 'button' is used to which the lens is blocked [Fig.19.1]. Alloys with low melting point ranging from about 47 to 85°C are used as the adhesive. It was a logical development to cast the button in alloy and block the lens to it in one operation. The alloy blocking machine consists of a reservoir for the metal, with a heater and one or more casting moulds, a means of controlling the flow and an ejector to remove the blocked on lens.

To ensure adhesion of the metal to the lens, a coating of lacquer is normally applied before blocking. A more recent innovation is to apply a plastics film supplied in rolls and coated on one side with an adhesive. The film is affixed by means of a vacuum operated applicator and then trimmed to size. Not only does this film give a good surface to take the metal but also at the cleaning stage it has merely to be peeled off.

Fig.19.1 Lens blocked for surfacing [H-pin location holes; B-button; A-Alloy; L-Lens]

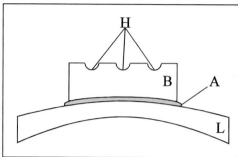

In the first stage of surfacing a generator is used and two basic forms are available, spherical and toroidal. Their purpose is to remove material quickly and to produce a good approximation of the surface required. The grinding element of a spherical generator is a diamond-impregnated lap, revolving at high speed, of the form referred to as a 'cup' or 'crown'. As shown in Fig.19.2, a cross-sectional diagram, it is a short tube with a relatively thin wall having a radius end. Such a tube would make a circular line of contact when applied to any part of a larger spherical surface. In any position of contact, the axis **ZZ** of the tube would necessarily pass through the centre of curvature **C** of the spherical surface.

Fig.19.2 Spherical generator set for convex surface

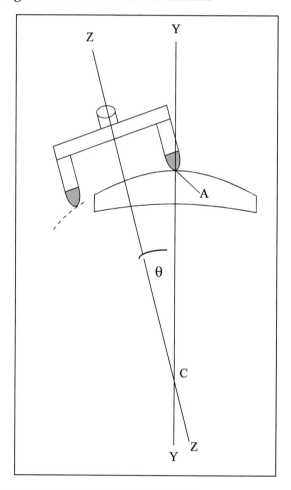

The lens is held in a chuck on a vertical spindle and slowly rotated about the axis **YY**. To produce a convex spherical surface, the lap is angled as in Fig.19.2 so that its axis of rotation **ZZ** makes an angle θ with the axis of revolution of the lens. The centre of curvature **C** lies at the intersection of these two axes. It will be evident that the radius of curvature of the surface is determined by the angle θ which is pre-set accordingly.

In order to grind the whole surface, the lap must be positioned as shown in Fig.19.3 so that the circle of contact passes through the vertex **A** of the surface, that is, its point of intersection with the axis of revolution **YY**.   As the lens rotates, every point on its surface will pass beneath the lap and be subjected to the grinding process.

Fig.19.3 Circle of contact between lap and lens

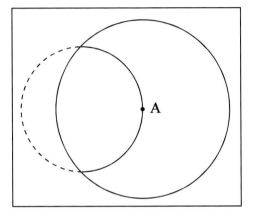

The arrangement for grinding a concave surface is shown in Fig.19.4. A plane surface is produced by setting the axis of revolution of the crown parallel to that of the lens.

Fig.19.4 A spherical generator set for concave surface

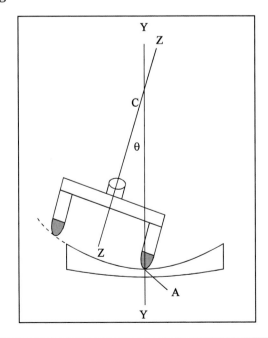

The toroidal surface has two different radii of curvature in its mutually perpendicular base and cross curve meridians. As will be seen by referring to Fig.5.1, illustrating the tyre and the barrel formation, it could be generated by a lap in the form of a disc with its centre of rotation at **C**, the lens blank being arced across it about the axis of rotation **OO′**. Alternatively, the lens blank could remain stationary and the rotating lap arced across it about the axis of revolution **OO′**. In principle, one or other of these systems is used in the toric generator.

By using a crown lap of the same type as in the spherical generator, a range of curves can be produced in one meridian. The mode of action can be followed from Fig.19.5 in which the lens blank must be imagined to be drawn across the lap in a straight line parallel to **XX**. The result would be to produce a concave curve of approximately cylindrical form with its axis parallel to **XX**. In fact the profile of the curve would be elliptical rather than circular because the projection of a tilted circle is an ellipse.

Now suppose the blank was arced across the lap by pivoting about an axis of revolution perpendicular to the plane of the diagram and passing through the point **C**. An approximately toroidal surface would be produced, of radius **CP** in the plane of the diagram.

Fig.19.5 Principle of the toric generator

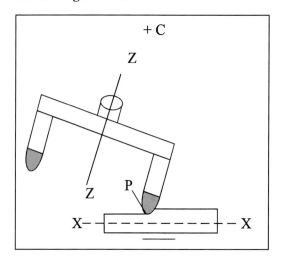

Smoothing has two different functions; to true the surface and to produce a surface capable of taking a good polish. By using various selected grades of abrasive and speed material is removed from the surface. Often both the tool and the lens are moved. In smoothing and polishing spherical lenses it is advantageous to have both tool and lens rotating, with one oscillating over the other as shown in Fig.19.6. The tool is rotated but there is no separate drive on the lens. The revolution of the tool imparts some rotational movement on the lens.

The following requirements must be met when smoothing and polishing astigmatic surfaces, particularly toroidal. This involves a much more complicated mechanism.

- The cylinder axis or base curve meridian of the lens must remain parallel to that of the tool during the whole of its travel. Some means of constraint is therefore essential.
- The relative motion of the tool and lens must ensure that the abrasive action is evenly distributed over the whole lens area.
- The actual path of the lens over the tool must not be too rapid or simply repetitive or there will be a tendency to produce a wavy pattern on the surface.
- The mechanical arrangement for imparting the separate motions of the lens and tool must be free from bias or misalignment tending to produce curvature errors.

Fig.19.6 General arrangement for smoothing and polishing spherical surfaces:
         L - lens;   T - tool

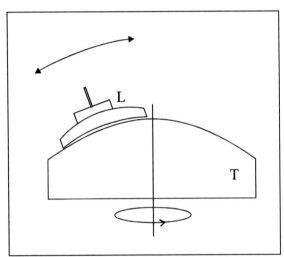

To obtain a good polished surface, a good smooth must be accomplished, resulting in a fine matt and even surface. Though polishing can be carried out on machines of the same design as those use for smoothing, variations in the stroke, pressure and running speeds may be necessary. Cerium oxides are usually employed in polishing slurry.

The lens must now be separated from its holder. One highly technical and sophisticated method is to give the block a sharp tap and in practised hands it is very effective. There is however a risk of breakage and, for that reason, melting off is generally favoured. Both the lens and block are immersed in water which is at a slightly higher temperature than the alloy's melting point.. Rinsing the lens and block before de-blocking is advisable.

All traces of any lacquer used must now be removed from the lens by using a suitable solvent. Obviously if a plastics film has been used this process is much cleaner and simpler. The lens is then cleaned thoroughly and dried.

The stages outlined above can be applied to any CR39 lenses which need to be surfaced, although there are certain differences which should be observed in the application of the processes. If the same tools are to be used for both glass and plastics then obviously compensations must be made for the difference in the refractive indices of the two types of material. It can be shown that for a different refractive index n', the tool would be:

$$(n - 1)F/(n' - 1)$$

The main problem to avoid when blocking is distortion of the lens by undue heat and lack of support. It is essential to use an alloy with a melting point at the lower end of the available range. The plastics film mentioned earlier gives better protection against heat transfer than lacquer, and cooling rings in the blocking unit are advisable to disperse the heat during the casting of the button. The diameter of the button should also be made as large as possible so as to give maximum support to the lens which is being processed.

Whereas the generating process is essentially the same as with glass and the removal material is fast, it is recommended that a number of smaller cuts are preferable to one larger one.

Smoothing of plastics lenses is usually two stages compared with the single one for glass. The maxim that a good polish demands a good smooth applies with particular force to plastics lenses.

When polishing it is vitally important that no abrasive emery or slurry is carried over from the smoothing process, hence both lens and tool must be well washed. A suspension of tin or aluminium oxide is used for polishing, the tool being faced with a velvety pad.

The same process as is used for glass is used for de-blocking, but considerably more care must be taken to avoid scratching of the surface.

Glazing is the operation of fitting lenses to a spectacle frame or mount although this term is usually understood to include the previous processes of *cutting* and *edging*. Cutting is the process of marking a slightly oversize outline of the desired shape on one surface of the uncut lens and removing the waste. Edging is the subsequent process of grinding the edge to produce the required finished size and shape, together with the desired edge form. The term applied to insertion of the edged lenses into a plastics frame is *springing in*.

In order to understand the range of equipment required to carry out glazing we need to look at the various tasks involved. If the work is to be carried out in a small workshop, or by the optician personally, the following stages are necessary to produce a glazed pair of single-vision lenses to a plastics or metal frame:

- Select suitable lenses from stock
- Check powers
- Mark optical centre and axis
- Select and measure frame
- Produce former[*or scan frame*]
- Lay off to correct decentration
- Check 'cut out'
- Block
- Auto edge
- Check size and fit
- Produce safety chamfer
- Fit lens
- Set up frame
- Check the finished spectacles

Before a lens can be edged it must be marked so that its cylinder axis [where applicable] is set as specified by the prescription and its optical centre is in the correct position. This process is known as *laying off*. It is possible to lay off a lens by the use of a simple protractor chart and marking pen, but is more accurately carried out using a focimeter or even a semi-automatic blocking machine. The reliability of any procedure of course is largely dependent upon the accuracy of the setting up of the equipment in the first place and also that of the operator.

When laying off by hand, the focimeter is used to mark the optical centre - often as a sequel to checking the power of the lens. Firstly, the axis line on the focimeter is set at the required prescription axis and the power scale at the combined power of the sphere and cylinder. If the prescription reads –4.50DS/+1.50DC x 70 for instance then the axis setting is at 70° and the power scale is –3.00D. The position of the lens is next adjusted until the target pattern is centralised on the screen or in the eyepiece. The marking device of the focimeter is then activated. The three dots showing the optical centre and horizontal meridian of the lens. If no decentration is called for, the uncut lens is merely placed with the marked optical centre directly over the centre of the protractor. The dots should, of course, be made to lie on the horizontal line of the protractor. If any decentration has been specified, then the lens must be placed on the protractor so that the marked centre is correspondingly displaced. Once this has been done then a horizontal line is marked across the front surface of the lens immediately above the horizontal line of the protractor and a short vertical line is also drawn. Figure 19.1 shows a lens with its axis at 70° laid off for the right eye so as to give a decentration of 2*mm* down and 3*mm* in. It is usual to denote the nasal edge of the horizontal line with an arrow head as shown, and in addition the lens is marked **R** or **L**.

One of the biggest drawbacks of glazing in a small workshop is the problem of storage and retrieval of the glazing former. Most larger frame manufacturers will supply formers with their products, but for all other frames, it is necessary to produce a former as and when required, which is time consuming. Finished formers have to be stored and retrieved from a library. Systematically numbering and keeping track of them is not an easy task.

Fig.19.1 Lens laid off for the right eye axis 70° [decentration *2mm* down and *3mm* in]

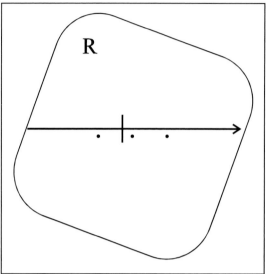

Modern technology has come to the rescue with electronic tracing of the frame shape which means that the need to store large numbers of formers has disappeared. When such formers are obtained from the manufacturers or suppliers, they are usually about 4*mm* to 5*mm* thick, having been produced directly from the master formers. This means they will not bend in use and this, combined with the basic accuracy of the shape, allows the user to produce a finished lens to fine tolerances.

Formers cut for individual frames however, are made from sheet material about 1*mm* to 2*mm* thick. This can bend in use, producing inaccurate shapes. It is also possible for the former cutting machine to 'stretch' frames with thin rims and, again, produce a distorted shape.

The latest electronic tracing machines overcome most of these problems. They are highly accurate, do not normally distort the frame [if used correctly] and the shape, once traced can often be stored in the system computer.

Most modern glazing systems use this method of shape selection and retrieval, allowing the shape to be recalled by the simple expedient of entering the job or shape number into a keypad or bar-code reader.

For blocking, the shape is displayed on a small screen, after which, centration details are entered. The screen then displays the optical centre, fitting cross or segment position as appropriate in the correct location. The uncut lens is then placed on a lens rest and the outline superimposed over the required finished shape. Any 'cut out' problems are obvious at this stage.

Once the correct position is found, the machine is used to block the lens, usually using an adhesive pad and re-useable holder. The lens is finally transferred to the auto-edger, where the shape details are retrieved again by entering the job or shape number. The previously stored data is then used to cut the required shape.

Some of the latest machines are also capable of tracing the cut lens shape using three-dimensional co-ordinates, as opposed to two-dimensional ones. The lens shape in Fig.19.2 shows that the lens size can be considered as the dimensions of the x-axis and the y-axis. Using these co-ordinates, the system can trace, plot and reproduce the lens shape on the screen for cutting purposes.

However these co-ordinates do not take into consideration the shape of the frame, which must be 'bowed' to allow for the curvature of the lens. This curvature, which occurs at 90° to the x-plane, is termed the z-axis and forms the third co-ordinate to complete the three-dimensional shape of the finished lens. Fig.19.3.

Fig.19.2

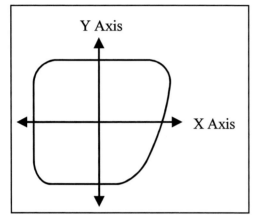

'Measuring' the curvature differences between the front and back surfaces at many points around the edge of the lens [along the z-axis] allows calculation of the variations in thickness around the periphery of the finished lens. This information can then be used to ensure that the bevel is correctly placed at all points around the lens periphery, allowing for exaggerated shapes, high cylinder powers and prism thickness.

Fig.19.3

Automatic placement of the bevel is another major advantage of the modern auto-edger, giving higher accuracy and reducing time wasted on having to manually place the bevel. All of this leads to the faster production of lenses which are right first time and require no subsequent hand finishing and re-shaping. The only drawback is the increase in cost due to the increased sophistication. These increases can be offset where the production levels are high.

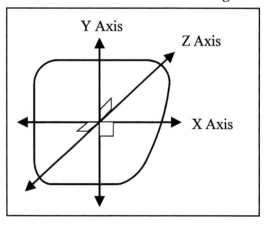

Most of the auto lens edgers on the market are designed for use with both glass and plastics lenses and, as such, make use of diamond wheels and water as the lubricant and coolant. Though edging machines run the entire gamut from the simple hand edger to the versatile electronic machines, the grinding agent is invariably a form of wheel although some designed for edging plastics lenses use a milling cutter. Edging wheels are of two types - grit and diamond - which are, nevertheless, similar in principle, the grinding being performed by particles of abrasive held in a bond of softer material.

Automatic flat edging and bevel edging machines have been known for many years. In all these machines the lens is mounted on a rotating spindle and held against the grinding surface of an abrasive wheel by gravity or spring pressure. The shape is controlled by the former. The rotation of the spindle can be controlled so as to eliminate unproductive time. Instead of rotating at uniform speed, the spindle is allowed to 'dwell' in one position as long as material is being removed. The various edging profiles can be incorporated in one machine as illustrated in Fig.19.4. This shows a Weco D111, with its normal grinding wheel combination for ordinary V-bevel, flat edge and mini-bevel, edges all medium powered and normal thin lenses.

Fig.19.4 Weco D111 grinding wheel

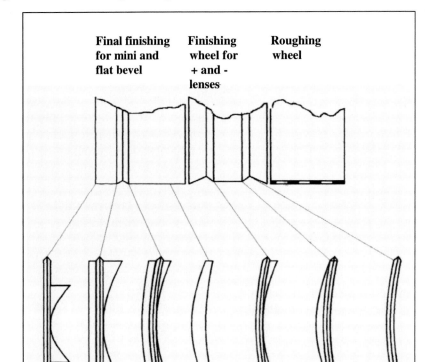

From the standpoint of glazing, rimmed spectacle frames are divided into 'metal' or 'plastics' and these are covered in greater detail in chapter 21. It would be generally agreed that plastics frames are the easier to glaze. One reason is that the lens size is not so critical since the rims are capable of being slightly stretched.

In glazing plastics frames, heat is usually required to soften the rims so that they can be eased over the edge of the lens, allowing the bevel to enter the groove. There are many different types of frame heater in operation today ranging from the simplest form of shell heater to automatic frame heaters with variable heat control for different frame weights. Many heaters incorporate a blower directing a stream of hot [or cold] air on to the frame. Sometimes a tank of heated glass beads is used.

Irrespective of the type of heater used it is essential that the frame should be softened sufficiently without it becoming scorched or blistered.

After glazing, when the frame has cooled, it should not be possible to rotate the lens in the rim by finger pressure alone, although in order to correct minor axis errors, a suitable pair of gripping pliers can often do the trick.

The traditional type of joint fitted to metal frames serves a double purpose, to close the rim about the lens, and to provide a means of attachment of the side. The latter should be able to pivot freely but should not be so loose that it can fall under its own weight. Although this type of joint is small and neat, it does require the lens size to be exact. If the lens is only slightly oversize the two halves of the joint will be forced apart, as shown in Fig.19.5, thus throwing an undue strain on the joint screw and tending to make the side loose. On the other hand, the lens should not be made undersize because it could be rotated in the rim or even dislodged. No gap should be visible at any point between the edge of the lens and metal eyewire

Fig.19.5 Traditional metal joint showing the effect of an oversize lens

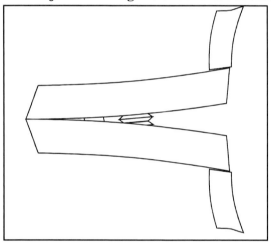

This traditional type of joint is now little used, and its place has largely been taken by other designs. One is the barrel joint consisting of a short tube attached to each free end of the eyewire. The joint screw passes through a clearance hole in one tube and engages in the other, which is threaded. Since the purpose of this construction is merely to close the rim, the spectacle sides require a separate means of attachment.

The block joint now in common use is attached to the upper end of the rim and has a recess which accommodates a short threaded tube or barrel soldered to the lower end of the rim. Another operation which may be necessary before inserting the lens is to 'bow' the eyewire to follow the peak of the bevel of the lens. The more the shape of a curved [meniscus or toric] lens departs from a circle, the more its edge wanders backwards and forwards from a frontal plane.

To counter the general tendency of joint screws to work loose, various expedients have been devised. For example, the barrel joint may have a second [grub] screw set at right angles into the side of the barrel so as to lock into the thread of the main screw. Sometimes a lock nut is fitted to the screw. Peening the end of the screw and splaying it after glazing is another method. A simple alternative is to apply a solution such as Loctite to the screw thread before insertion.

The glazing of nylon supra mounts calls for a means of grooving the edge of the lens. The type of machine devised for this purpose uses a thin wheel with a diamond impregnated edge and incorporates a mechanical drive for steering the lens so that the groove remains central despite variations in edge thickness.

In rimless mounts, which are of various different types, the lens is held in position by a screw or screws passing through it or by claws engaging in small slots in the edge. Drilling a hole in a thin piece of glass is obviously a very tricky operation, to say nothing of the fact that breakages are expensive. Experience has shown that drilling a hole in one operation is too risky because of the probability of fracturing the lens when the drill breaks through the second surface of the lens. It is consequently standard practice to drill in two stages. The hole is started on one side and the drill allowed to penetrate just over half way. The lens is then turned over and the drilling completed from the other side. After drilling, the edges of the holes should be chamfered. Screws should not of course be over tightened and the ends should be neatly finished off by careful filing down taking care to damage neither the gold skin of the mount nor the lens.

20. SPECTACLE FRAME MATERIALS

Over the years a wide variety of materials have been used for making spectacle frames - wood. Leather, bone, horn, ivory, tortoiseshell and of course both base and precious metals such as steel, nickel aluminium, silver, gold and platinum.

None of these materials, other than metal has survived the advent of plastics, which burst in on the frame making industry 60 years ago. It had the good fortune to arrive at a time when tortoiseshell and horn were in full fashion but these materials were expensive and scarce so mottled plastics took over as the poor man's tortoiseshell.

Today, plastics materials satisfy the bulk of the frame market, although metal frames are once again increasing in popularity and indeed they seem to dominate men's styling.

Materials used in the production of spectacle frames need to possess certain important properties and plastics have been found to have just those required for producing frames that are both practical and good-looking. Important properties are:
- Ease of production
- Dermatitic compatibility
- Dimensional stability
- Colour fastness
- Mechanical durability

Other virtues possessed by plastics are:
- low specific gravity
- good strength/weight ratio
- good electrical and thermal insulation
- high resistance to chemicals

Plastics are materials which essentially consist of macromolecular organic compounds produced either synthetically or by the transformation of natural materials Macromolecules [polymers] are formed in great numbers of largely identical basic components [monomers] which are linked together by polymerisation, polycondensation or polyaddition. The raw materials for fully synthetic plastics are petroleum, natural gas, coal etc.; those for transformed natural products are cellulose, protein, natural rubber and resins.

Those suitable for the manufacture of frames fall roughly into five groups: *cellulose nitrate; cellulose acetate;* [including butyrates and propionates]; *acrylics; nylons and epoxy resins*.

The macromolecules are held together by chemical and/or physical binding forces, which results in the following classification.

- **Thermoplastics** - which consist of physically combined macromolecules. They are solid or visco-elastic at room temperature and can be shaped and reshaped repeatedly by heating without chemical transformation. In thermoplastics, linear macromolecules may be evenly arranged in parallel and form crystallites, which are visible under the microscope. A structure lacking any kind of order is called amorphous. Thermoplastics are meltable, weldable and soluble. All the materials used in the manufacture of plastics spectacle frames fall into this category.

- **Thermosetting** - such plastics consist of chemically closely combined macromolecules. Physical binding forces are also active. Thermosetting plastics are usually very hard and brittle at room temperature. They are heat resistant, are not re-shapeable, meltable, weldable or soluble.

Most plastics can be sawn, blanked, milled, buffed and barrelled successfully, thus lending themselves to either hand or mass production processing. Some of the operations can be carried out while the material is cold, but some heat is required for blanking, coring temples or inserting pinless hinges.

The ease with which these materials can be manipulated brings joy to the optician who is called upon to make final adjustments to the frame fitting. All he or she needs is a good frame heater, a few pliers and experience.

It is obviously important that the material chosen for a frame should have no harmful effects on the skin, and in this respect plastics have a very safe record. Although isolated cases of allergy do occur, discomfort from a frame is more likely from bad fitting than from any chemical reaction. Whilst it is important that the plastics should not affect the skin, it is equally important that the wearer's body acids do not attack the plastics. Some plastics will craze and embrittle more quickly than others, particularly if they are worn at extreme temperatures.

No plastics can have the strength of a metal frame but most are reasonably durable and some, like nylon, are almost unbreakable. A new very tough material called carbon-X has recently been introduced; it is a mixture of nylon and carbon fibre and is more fully described under nylon materials.

Since the purpose of the frame is to hold the lenses, its dimensional stability should be approaching that of glass. In this respect plastics is inferior to metal, but since plastics can be worked within fractions of a millimetre, when accurately glazed they are capable of withstanding any extremes of temperature.

It is well known that certain dyes are more fugitive than others and that the degree of colour stability will vary with the type of plastics used and the colour of the dye required. Pearls, pinks and pale blues seem to be most vulnerable, but the problem has been largely overcome with the new extruded acetate materials that have a good record for colour retention.

Cellulose is a naturally occurring polymer derived from wood pulp and cotton linters and the family of cellulostic plastics is produced by a variety of chemical modifications. Although it is not itself a thermoplastic, it can be made into a whole range of thermoplastics such as cellulose nitrate, cellulose acetate, cellulose triacetate, cellulose butyrate or propionate - all of which, with the exception of triacetate, are used in the production of spectacle frames.

Cellulose nitrate - the first cellulose derivative used commercially was a cellulose nitrate called Celluloid; it was patented in 1869 and was used for spectacle frames very successfully, indeed for more than half a century it dominated the frame business as it has all the properties required of a frame material - toughness, dimensional stability, surface lustre etc. Unfortunately it is highly inflammable and, in the 1950s a safety conscious public began to outlaw it and although in some countries it is not officially banned, its use has dwindled to near extinction as new types of much tougher cellulose acetates have been introduced.

Cellulose acetates - These are the plastics most widely used in spectacle frame manufacture and the materials are made by hydrolysing cellulose triacetate to remove some of the acetyl groups. In production the cellulose polymer is steeped in acids, made into solid form and then ground into a powder. At the plastics producing works this powder is mixed with a solvent, a plasticiser and various pigments and, after stirring and kneading, it emerges with the consistency of pure rubber and is known as 'dough'.

After filtering the 'dough' is rolled into sheets on heavy metal plates and pressed into blocks. These are sometimes sliced down at various angles to produce attractive colour effects. To make extruded strip, the powder is mixed with a plasticiser and then forced out of a nozzle to produce strips of different and varied dimensions. Some acetate sheets have a laminated colour on top of the sheet. By chamfering the top surface of the frame, various effects can be obtained, such as two-tone or colour flashes at the temples. Extrusion opens up a completely new field of colour design possibilities as well as producing a tougher and more satisfactory material. Acetate is a thermoplastic. This means that it softens when heated, but doesn't burn like nitrate, although it will blister if overheated. It is easy to work with, though care must be taken not to overheat or 'roll' the rims when fitting lenses.

Fig.20.1 Acetate sheet

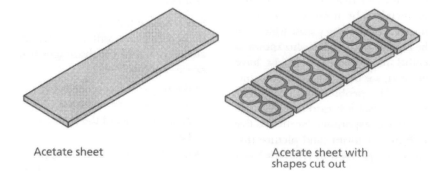

Acetate sheet

Acetate sheet with shapes cut out

Fig.20.2 Laminated sheet

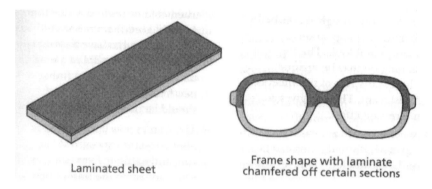

Laminated sheet

Frame shape with laminate
chamfered off certain sections

Cellulose propionate - This material is made by substituting propionic acid for cellulose triacetate and this results in a material which is gaining increased popularity on account of its greater strength, higher temperature resistance, greater elasticity and greater resistance to ageing. Moreover propionate frames are lighter in weight than acetate frames of the same volume. A further reduction in weight can be obtained by the use of thinner material.

One reason propionate frames have been slow to take on is the fact that they are produced by a moulding process, and as moulds are costly tools to make, frame styling must be limited to those designs in which sculpturing and decorative features are an integral part of the mould.

Cellulose propionate is also a thermoplastic and similar to acetate in the way that it behaves. Because it is moulded, though, as well as being made thinner, it tends to hold its shape better, because it doesn't 'remember' a flat state.

Similarly with *nylon*, the manufacturing process is carried out by moulding, but in this case injection moulding must be used and the high cost of these tools and the capital cost of equipment can only be economically justified when enormous quantities of a single item are required. Nylon production is usually limited therefore to sunglasses and safety eyewear. It is a first-generation polyamide. It is generally considered to be of poor appearance. It is difficult to fit and adjust, but is strong and flexible.

Polyamide is a new type of moulded plastic material, produced in much the same way as propionate. It doesn't, however, have plasticisers like acetate and propionate, but it does have a mechanical stability which allows it to keep its shape even with the rim as thin as 1.3*mm*. It is a member of the nylon family and known by other names depending upon the manufacturer (e.g. Charmant 'Polyflex' and Silhouette 'SPX'). Polyamide is lightweight and can be made even thinner than propionate. This allows very thin-rimmed plastic frames to be made, some so thin they need reverse bevels, requiring the lenses to be grooved just like supra or nylon-cord frames. This works well with minus prescriptions since the flat edge minimises the power 'rings'.

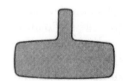

Fig.20.3 Profile view of reverse bevel

Carbon fibre is the new material which is being used in the carbon-X range. It is an extremely strong and lightweight material being used extensively in sports equipment, dinghies, aircraft etc., and the carbon-X material used for spectacles consists of 60% nylon and 20% carbon fibre. Because the frames are injection moulded, the styling and colour range are somewhat limited, although their strength makes them virtually unbreakable. They have a fibre or whisker (potassium titanate) mixed in with a flexible nylon compound. Because these whiskers can be visible, carbon fibre frames are always solid colours. They are also fitted cold because they do not respond well to heat.

In the 1960s a new frame material appeared on the scene; it was made by the Austrian frame makers, Wilhelm Anger, and its name *'Optyl'* became known throughout the world for its distinctive property and its high styling. Optyl is made from thermoplastic epoxy resin mixed with selected hardeners and requires no plasticisers. Its physical properties show many promising advantages over other materials. Compression moulding techniques are the only production methods used for this material.

Moulding increases tooling costs on short runs and inhibits style changes but, on the other hand, greater flexibility in stock control is enjoyed because the frames are moulded in clear material and this enables the frames to be stocked and finished later to whatever colour effect is required by the customer.

To the frame manufacturer, Optyl brought about a big reduction in material wastage, since up to 85% of acetate sheet may end up as unusable waste; a further advantage to the manufacturer is the ease with which three-dimensional sculpted effects and complex cut-outs can be produced by moulding.

To the optician, glazing and manipulation of the finished frame present the same type of problem as found in acrylic, but Optyl material has a high and attractive lustre which is more resistant to body acids, colour fast, light in weight and is amongst the hardest plastics materials used for spectacle frames.

In the days when colonial settlers were kitted out with topees and khaki drill for service in the tropics, they always included in their kit a pair of *solid gold* spectacles which could resist constant immersion in perspiration expected in the steamy jungle. Although the precaution was not entirely unnecessary, solid gold spectacles have now gone the way of the topee, and other modern metals can be trusted to give good service under any climatic conditions.

There is still today a small but thriving market for solid gold and this may be expected to grow as metal styles generally increase in popularity. Although legally described as solid gold, i.e. 24 carat, as this metal would be too soft for frame making, as well as being too expensive, they are not in fact made of pure gold.

As used in the jewellery and spectacle trades, solid carat gold is actually an alloy in which copper and silver are mixed with the gold to make up its 24 parts - thus 24*ct.* gold is pure gold, 18*ct.* gold has 18 parts pure and 6 parts alloy and in 12*ct.* gold, only half the metal is pure gold.

Rolled gold or, as the Americans call it, gold-filled is produced by bonding a skin of carat gold on to a core of base metal, usually nickel silver and other metals such as manganese silver, bronze, tin etc., may be used. The gold-filled block then undergoes a series of cold hammering and rolling until it is the size suitable for being drawn into frame making wire, when it is again beaten into final form by huge machines using high-speed rotary hammers. The gold-filled wire is then sold to the frame makers in large rolls and is already profiled for eyerims and other component parts.

Frames are stamped to indicate the total gold content of a frame - thus   1/10 12*ct*. which would indicate that the 12*ct*. gold content accounts for 1/10th of the total weight of the frame. An alternative way of expressing the gold content is used in many countries where it is shown in parts per 1000 of total weight - thus 1/20 10*ct*. equals 20 parts per thousand and 1/10 12*ct*. equals 50 parts per thousand, often stamped ⑤⓪ . Most countries have very strict laws to regulate the stamping of gold articles.

A major change in metal frame making has taken place in the last 20 years. The soaring cost of pure gold has made gold-filled stock material a risky investment and fewer frame manufacturers are prepared to hold stocks of this costly item. The same problem, in a more serious form has been experienced in the jewellery trade which fortunately had the resources with which to research and develop alternative multi-layer coatings which were equally durable but more economical than the use of pure gold. Different types of multi-layered coatings have been tried - for instance a thin layer of platinum has been found to provide a successful anti-corrosion barrier after which a thin film of pure gold can be used; this and other forms of gilding are now being used extensively on spectacle frames

There are six metals used in the platinum group; ruthenium [Ru], rhodium [Rh], palladium [Pd], osmium [Os], iridium [Ir] and platinum [Pt]. The hardness of platinum can be doubled by the addition of iridium.

Titanium is a very light, strong material, although also very expensive. It is about 40% lighter than other metals used in the manufacture of spectacle frames. Unlike gold it cannot be soldered.

Titanium is a metallic element which, following aluminium, iron and manganese, ranks fourth in abundance among the earth's elements. It was as recently as 1948 that DuPont first produced the metal for general use, for it had been found in the space industries, marine and nuclear power industries and many others, that its unique properties are of value. It has attracted the spectacle frame maker because it is:
- lightweight - it has a specific gravity of $4.5g/cm^3$ which makes it only about half the weight of nickel silver.
- flexible - its elasticity factor is 20% higher than that of nickel silver.
- corrosion resistant - higher than that of gold or nickel silver.
- abrasion resistant - its surface hardness is three times greater than rolled gold and ten times greater than gold plated frames.

The manufacture of spectacle frames in titanium involves many problems in cutting, pressing, soldering and finishing and entirely new plating methods have to be used. The result is that the finished product is relatively costly.

Nowadays, the components of a high quality metal frame are made of a wide variety of alloys to meet the partly conflicting demands which are made of it, e.g. elasticity is required of the sides, torsional strength of the lens rims and stability of the bridge. It was above all the introduction of electroplating which made this procedure possible. Table 20.1 shows some of the alloys used today along with their most important properties.

Soldering consists of the joining of metallic materials below their melting temperature. The solders necessary for this process are metal alloys or pure metals. Soft solders require a working temperature of under 450°C, hard solders a temperature in excess of this. Solders often contain flux consisting of a non-metallic substance to ensure that the solder covers the surfaces to be joined.

In hard soldering the junction points between the parts to be bonded are heated to at least the melting range of the solder, or the temperature of the parts to be bonded lies slightly above the melting temperature of the solder. Capillary action forces the liquid solder into the slit separating the parts, the solder then diffuses into the surface of the material and thus creates a permanent bond.

Table 20.1 Properties and applications of major alloys for spectacle frames

Material [alloy]	Density [g/cm^3]	Melting point [°C]	Corrosion resistance	Solder-ability	Weld-ability	Use
rolled gold			very good	very good		all components
pure nickel	8.9	1455	very good	good	good	pad arms
German silver Cu,Ni,Zn	8.62 - 8.71	950 - 1025	satisfactory	very good	good	hinges, decoration
Monel Cu,Ni,Zn,Sn	8.8	1046	satisfactory	good	good	sides, bridges
bronze Cu,Sn	8.86	865	satisfactory	good	very good	closing blocks

In welding the parts to be joined are molten and bonded homogeneously with each other by the application of pressure via electrodes. In the case of larger surfaces, e.g. joints/sides, the homogeneous bonding is usually restricted to preformed projections especially made for this purpose. A prerequisite for this type of welding without the use of filler materials is that the parts to be bonded must display identical or very similar melting temperatures.

Electroplating is a process for coating the surface of metallic objects by the electrolytic and chemical deposition of a metal covering. It is used for gold and chromium plating of metal spectacle frames which are suspended in a specially compounded bath [electrolyte].

Fig.20.1 Principle of electroplating

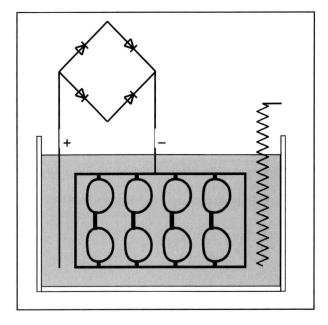

The major components of an electrolyte for gold plating are gold, copper, palladium, sulphides, cyanides and phosphates in the form of dissolved salts and additives such as glossing and wetting agents, with distilled water as the solution carrier. The contents are mixed in an exactly defined ratio in the solution carrier. Alloy baths in 18 or 22 carat are used, with the alloys being deposited with the gold in the mixed crystal. This is of decisive importance for resistance to corrosion and tarnishing.

In [white] chromium plating, chromium, an element of exceptional hardness with a bluish white hue and high brilliance, is deposited for the purpose of corrosion protection on a layer of pure nickel using an electroplating process.

In black chromium plating, metallic chromium and chromium-VI-oxide are deposited in a certain ratio using high current densities and exact temperature cycles. This results in a dull black coating which is given its finish by immersion in a special emulsion.

Electrostatic powder coating is now used in many areas of the metal industry as a method of coating materials with plastics. The wet coating process which was formerly also practised for spectacle frames has certain drawbacks with regard to adhesive strength and has therefore been replaced by electrostatic powder coating.

This process uses the principle of electrostatic charging. The powder is swirled in a container and conveyed to a spray gun, at the exit aperture of which it is then charged by means of electrolytes. At the same time, a strong electrostatic field is built up between the exit aperture and the stand holding the spectacle frames. The powder particles are then attracted by the frames due to the charge and the electrostatic field, and adhere to their surface. The mount holding the frames rotates during the spraying process, and the spray gun moves up and down at a set rhythm, ensuring uniform powdering of the entire surface of the frames.

For dyeing, a layer of powder is first applied to the frames. The powder particles are then melted in a circulating-air oven at relatively high temperatures until they form a transparent, clear coating of plastics, after which they are then dyed using the infiltration process. Different colour concentration and tones are possible with this process by varying the length of immersion periods. Graduated tones and multicolour effects can be achieved by using a succession of different dye baths.

The so-called coloured gold coating is a combination of electroplating and electrostatic powder coating. A multilayer electroplating process is also used here, but only for colouring purposes. The plastics coating then performs the function of sealing the layers of gold, providing a sufficient degree of scratch and corrosion resistance.

At one period during the development of fashion frames, great hopes were placed on the use of aluminium and many styles were successfully introduced. The metal is stain and tarnish resistant, is durable, light in weight and can be anodised in attractive colours. The big disadvantage to the frame makers was the fact that it could not be soldered or brazed and had to be assembled by machining or riveting.

Aluminium is strong and very rigid and, although the frames proved durable in wear, their rigidity caused problems in glazing and adjusting. Aluminium frames have a characteristic bold, solid and rigid look, excellent for sunglass styling where glazing and adjustment problems are less important.

21. FRAME MEASUREMENTS

The measuring system for spectacle frames is based on the boxing system which uses a rectangle [or box] as the basis for the determination of the dimensions. It comprises several horizontal and vertical dimensions and reference points. The knowledge of these is necessary for the manufacturing, ordering and adjustment of spectacle frames as well as for the exact mounting of lenses into frames.

The following diagrams show the basic reference points for a spectacle frame.

Fig.21.1 Reference points for the measurement of a spectacle frame front

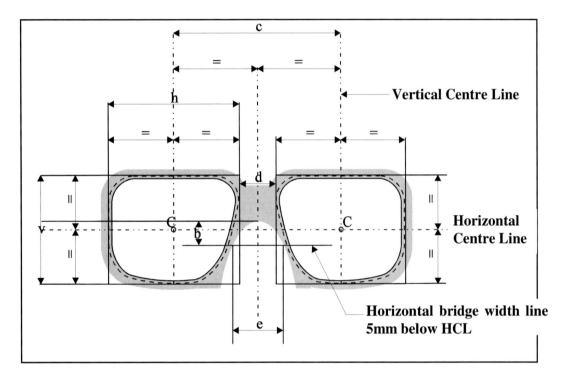

Fig.21.2 Dimensions for a drop-end side

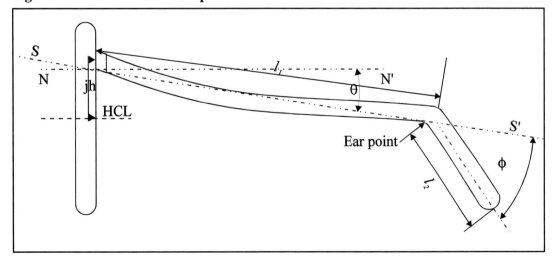

Fig.21.3 Dimensions for a curl side

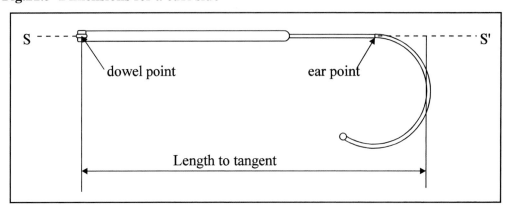

Table.21.1 Reference points and definitions

Reference	Term	Definition
C	Boxed centre	Intersection of the horizontal and vertical centre lines of the rectangular box containing the lens shape.
h	Horizontal lens size	Distance between the vertical sides of the rectangle containing the lens shape.
v	Vertical lens size	Distance between the horizontal sides of the rectangle containing the lens shape.
c	Distance between centres	Distance between the boxed centres 'C' [See Fig.21.1].
d	Distance between lenses	Distance between the nearest points of the apices of the two lenses.
l	Overall length of side	Length from the dowel point to the extreme end of the side [$l = l_1 + l_2$ see Fig.21.2].
l_1	Length to bend	Length from the dowel point and the ear point
l_2	Length to drop	Length from the ear point to the extreme end of the side.
e	Bridge width	Minimum distance between the pad surfaces of the frame measured along the bridge width line.
b	Bridge height	Vertical distance from the bridge width line to the mid-point of the lower edge of the bridge.

Horizontal Centre Line - This is a line drawn through the geometric centres of the rectangular boxes that just encompass the two lenses [Fig.21.1].

Angle of side - The vertical angle between a normal to the back plane of the front and the line of the side when opened [θ in Fig.21.2].

Frame temple width - Distance between the sides 25*mm* behind the back plane of the front [TW - Fig.21.4]

Frame head width - Distance between the sides at the ear points [HW - Fig.21.4].

Crest height - The vertical distance from the horizontal centre line to the mid-point of the lower edge of the bridge [Note the difference between this and the bridge height which is measured from the *bridge width line*].

Bridge projection [or inset] - Minimum horizontal distance from the back plane of the front to the centre of the back of the bridge [**p** & **i** Fig.21.5].

Bridge apical radius - The radius of the arc forming the lower edge of the bridge viewed perpendicularly to the back plane of the front [Fig.21.7].

Distance between rims [**DBR**] - The horizontal distance between the nasal surfaces of the rims [**b**] measured at a stated distance [**x**] below the mid-point of the lower edge of the bridge [Fig.21.8].

Splay angle of pad - Angle between the pad plane and a normal to the back plane of the front [**s** Fig.21.9].

Frontal angle of pad - Angle between the vertical and the line of intersection of the pad plane with the back plane of the front [**f** Fig.21.9].

Joint height - The distance from the centre line to the horizontal plane through the centre of the joint [**jh** Fig.21.2].

Length to tangent - The distance from the dowel point to a tangent to the inner surface of the curl [at rest] which is perpendicular to the line of the side [Fig.21.3].

Downward angle of drop - Downward inclination of the drop from the line of the side, measured near the ear point and in the vertical plane containing the line of the side [ϕ Fig.21.2].

Inward angle of drop - Inward inclination of the drop near the ear point from the vertical plane containing the line of the side [Fig.21.10].

Ear point - The mid-point of the arc of the bend of the side [Fig.21.2 - drop-end side]& and the point of the lower edge of the side at the beginning of the curl [Fig.21.3 - curl side].

Line of the side - A straight line through the dowel point and the ear point [**SS´** Fig.21.2].

Normal to the back plane of front - [**NN´** Fig.21.2].

Angle of let-back - Horizontal angle between the inner surface of the fully opened side, adjacent to the joint, and a normal to the back plane of the front [Fig.21.4].

Fig.21.4 Frame temple width, frame head width and angle of let-back

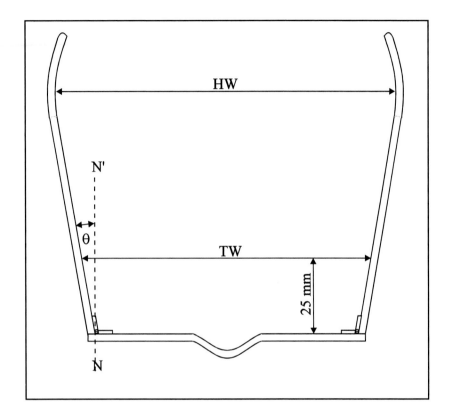

Fig.21.5 Bridge projection [or inset]   **Fig.21.6 Crest height**

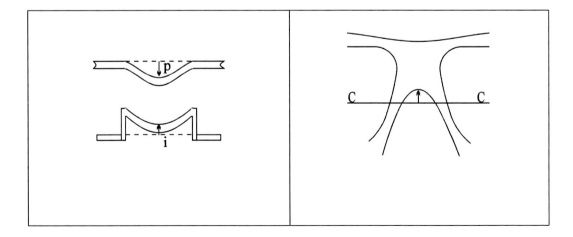

Fig.21.7 Apical radius

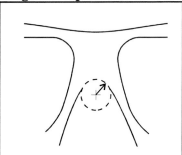

Fig.21.8 Distance between rims

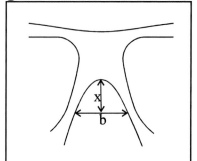

Fig.21.9 Pad angles

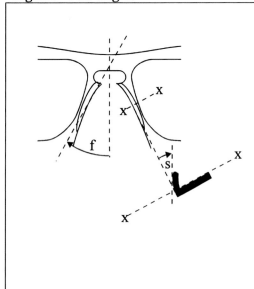

Fig.21.10 Inward angle of drop

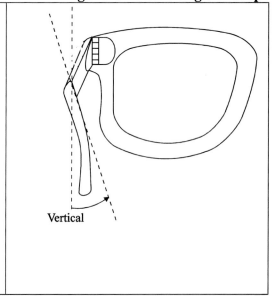

22. ADJUSTMENTS

The adjustment of spectacle frames is really something that can only be learned by practice. It is all very well to talk about the softening temperature of a particular plastics material as so many degrees centigrade, but so much is dependent upon the age of the frame, always assuming that the material has been correctly identified in the first place. What temperature does a particular frame heater achieve? The practical answers are that you must find out how far you can go with any individual frame by trial and error. It is inevitable that, at some stage, you will break or damage a frame whilst you are carrying out an adjustment, therefore it is probably a good idea to practise on old frames, odd sides etc. This should reduce the risk of calamities with a patient's new [or more likely old deeply loved and probably irreplaceable] frame.

First impressions are very important both in meeting people and in the fitting of a pair of spectacles. The following guidelines serve to illustrate how to achieve comfort and satisfaction for everybody by the proper adjustment of frames when they are initially collected, and also when they are re-adjusted following a period of wear.

Some opticians adopt a procedure of 'setting up' spectacles at the checking stage prior to advising the patient that they are ready for collection. Although the previous chapter dealt with a comprehensive list of measurements that can be taken for a spectacle frame and the next chapter will deal as fully with the ordering of the same, it is unfortunately often the case that precious few details are actually written on an order. It is my personal view therefore that unless the frame is grossly distorted, in which case return to the prescription house might be in order, then adjustment or setting up is best left until it can be judged on the patient's face.

This course of action does however mean that the optician should never hand the spectacles to the patient, but should begin the fitting procedure by putting the frame on the patient's face in the first instance. Thus if the frame is in need of some additional adjustment the optician will be instantly aware of this and can remove the frame immediately ensuring that the wearer is unaware of the fact and so does not become unnecessarily concerned that the glasses may not be correct. The wearer will not assume the adjustment is complete until the fitter hands over the frame to put it on for himself. If that is the first move, then a person's psychological reaction tends to be that the spectacles are ready, and any subsequent adjustments may be interpreted as an attempt to rectify an error and may lessen confidence in the 'fit'. You want that first impression to be a lasting one.

In order to place the spectacles on the wearer, they should be held by the sides, pulling slightly outwards to facilitate slipping the glasses on more easily, and guide the ends of the sides just over the ear point and then gently push them down. If you find that the sides must be spread out a good deal to get them on then you will probably need to increase the let back of the sides by filing the butt portion of each side until they open wide enough to permit the frame to rest on the nose without lateral pressure to the sides.

Triangle of force

The fitting triangle is shown in Fig.22.1 and is comprised of the three points where the spectacles contact or put pressure against the head. The apex of the triangle is the pressure point which is situated on the crest of the nose, and the base of the triangle is a line joining the two pressure points just above the ear points, one on each side of the head.

Where the frame has nose pads then there will actually be two resting points forming the apex of the triangle.

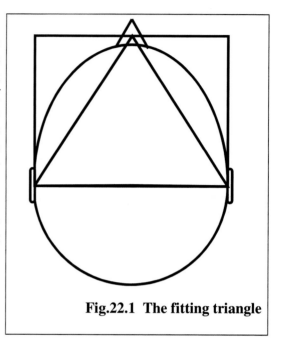

Fig.22.1 The fitting triangle

Let-back

The angle of let-back of the sides should be such that the sides exert no pressure, even if touching, on any area of the face or side prior to the point of the head where they should exert pressure - just above the root of the ears which is usually at the widest point of the head.

If the sides have not been let back far enough there will be too much pressure on both sides of the head, which, apart from the discomfort to the wearer, causes the sides to bow out as shown in Fig.22.2. This forces the frame forward until the sides are opposite a narrower part of the head and the pressure is somewhat relieved as in Fig.22.3. If the spectacles are fitted in this manner, without letting back the sides correctly, they will not only tend to slide down, but as they do so, the drop end of the sides will pull against the backs of the wearer's ears.

The result of all this is that the wearer experiences the disadvantages of both loose and tight glasses. That is they slip down the nose as well as hurt behind the ears.

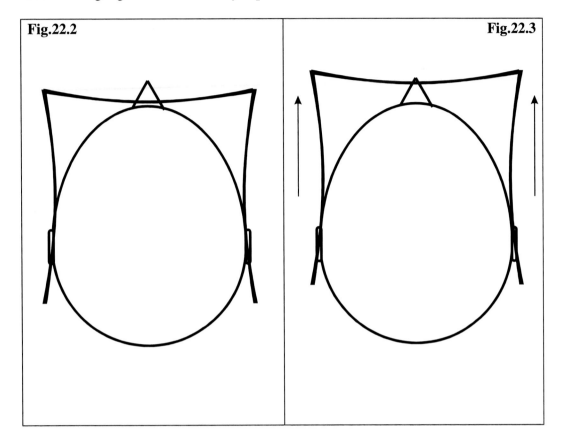

Fig.22.2   **Fig.22.3**

Equality of Lens Vertex Distance

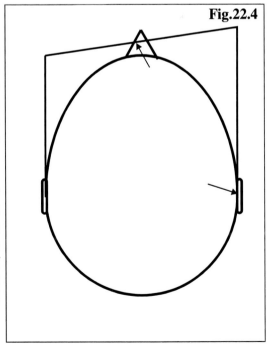

Fig.22.4

At this point it is advisable to check the spectacles on the patient's face in order to ascertain that the vertex distance of both lenses is equal. This can easily be carried out by requesting the wearer to tilt his head forward enabling you to view the spectacles from above [Fig.22.4].

If the glasses have been properly aligned and the wearer's head is symmetrical, then the vertex distances will be equal. If however the sides have been let-back by unequal amounts or if one side of the wearer's head is somewhat wider than the other, then the result will be inequality of the vertex distances.

The necessary procedures for correcting this inequality will be directly indicated by the manner in which the frame positions itself. If as in Fig.22.4 the right lens is further from the face than the left lens, there will be more pressure over the right ear than the left, forcing the right side out. The remedial action can be tackled in two ways.

- It may be that the right side is not let-back far enough, making this side fit too tight. The solution is to let the side back farther.

- It could also be that the right side is correctly fitted, but the let-back of the left side is too great. The right only has the effect of pushing its side forward due to the lack of counterbalancing pressure on the left side. The solution therefore is to bring this left side inward, decreasing the spread.

In practice, often both sides are adjusted somewhat, one being brought in, the other opened out. As stated previously, regardless of whether the problem lies with the spectacles or with the shape of the head, the solution is identical. If steps are not taken to alleviate this problem, then after being worn for some time the glasses will cause the ear on one side and the opposite side of the wearer's nose to become sore. As a result of this, if a person complains of the frame hurting on one side of the nose, an improper side let-back may be suspected. You should also note that when approaching the problem of vertex distance inequality, it is a good idea initially to check whether one of the sides is bowed in or out, and if so straighten it first. A single bowed side can cause a vertex distance inequality in the same way as differences in the let-back of the sides.

The Front.

Any adjustments to the frame front can be carried out after the let-back of the sides has been undertaken. Firstly the correct pantoscopic angle or tilt of the frame front is set and the straightness of the frame on the patient's face, when viewed from the front, is adjusted. It should be obvious that proper pantoscopic tilt and frame straightness needs to precede any bridge adjustments, since changes in the angle of the front will directly affect the seating of the nose-pads. If the nose-pads are made to sit flat on the nose and then the whole frame front is re-angled, a problem has been created - the pads will no longer be sitting flat on the nose.

Pantoscopic Angle.

The usual inclination of the front may vary anywhere between 0° and 20° from the vertical, varying to the upper extreme or more in the case of exceptionally protruding eyebrows. The lenses should touch neither the brows nor the cheeks. The pantoscopic tilt permits the optical axis to pass through the eye's centre of rotation. A rule of thumb is that, for each millimetre the optical centre is below the pupil centre, with the eye in the primary position, the pantoscopic angle should be increased by about 2°.

Frame Straightness in Wear

Adjustment of the angle of the side permits levelling of the frame as viewed from the front. Most heads are not symmetrical, and one ear is often slightly higher than the other. Where this occurs, perfectly trued glasses with parallel sides will result in a vertical discrepancy of the lenses with respect to each other when the sides rest on top of the ear points. Another possible cause of a crooked frame is when the sides are not angled equally. The solution again is the same whether the cause is the frame or the face. If the right side is too high, the right side must be angled up. This allows the frame to drop down farther on that side before the side contacts the top of the ear.

It may be inadvisable to decrease the angle of the higher side, as the frame front may then have insufficient tilt when viewed from the side. If that is the case the opposite side may be angled down. This increase in the angle of tilt of the opposite side accomplishes the same result as before by raising the side that is too low. If large changes in tilt are required it is often preferable to angle one side up and the other down in order to lessen the stress on the joints and also balance the appearance of the spectacles. The result of any adjustment to the side angles is that when the glasses are placed on a flat surface such as a table the wearer will be suspicious of the accuracy of the fitting of the frame until the quite normal asymmetries of his face are tactfully pointed out. Side angle should always be checked with spectacles this way ⌐╱not ⌐╲ in case length to bend and/or drop are different for right and left.

One further point to be wary of is if the sides have been angled by different amounts and the front appears straight when viewed from the front, it is possible that lenses do not have equal pantoscopic tilts because of a twist at the centre of the bridge. Again this should have been spotted and rectified before progressing with side angle adjustments.

Bridge Adjustment

Adjustments to the width of a bridge of a plastics frame are rarely carried out in practice at this stage. If fairly major adjustment is required in order to obtain a satisfactory fit, then it usually preferable to choose a frame with the correct bridge fitting at the dispensing stage. If the frame has adjustable pads or pads on arms the various modifications can be made in order to achieve a satisfactory fit.

Increasing the distance between the pads may be appropriate in cases when:
- the frame is too high on the face
- the segments or fitting crosses are too high
- the bridge is too small a fitting for the nose
- the vertex distance of the lenses is too great

Decreasing the distance between the pads would be appropriate in cases when:
- the frame sits too low on the face
- the segments or fitting crosses are too low
- the bridge is too large for the nose
- the lenses are sitting too close to the eyes and lashes

Vertex Distance

There are times when it is felt necessary to alter the vertex distance of the lenses. This type of alteration might be required if, for instance the top of the frame were resting against the brows or the bottom eyerim touching the cheeks and neither could be remedied by a change of side angle. Increasing the vertex is also needed as stated above when the eyelashes brush against the back surface of the lenses.

Decreasing the vertex distance, or bringing the frame closer to the face may be required for purely cosmetic reasons. It will also provide a wider field of corrected vision. For the bifocal wearer, moving the frame and lenses closer to the face increases the field of view above the bifocal without the need to lower the segment. This effect can also be produced by an increase in the pantoscopic angle. When high-powered lenses are involved, precise vertex measurement becomes very important. In some instances small alterations in the vertex distance of the finished spectacles may affect vision profoundly, especially with aspheric lenses

Fig.22.5 Examples of pliers

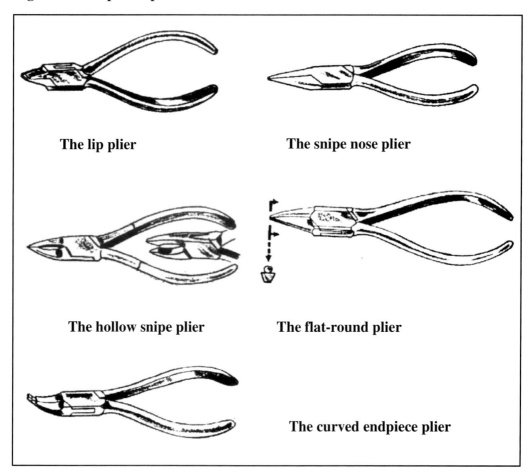

The lip plier   The snipe nose plier

The hollow snipe plier   The flat-round plier

The curved endpiece plier

The first item to be checked is to determine the presence or the absence of an "**X'd**" condition of the rims. This is a situation where the plane of one rim is at an angle to the plane of the other [Fig.22.6]. At first, one may be inclined to think that the rims arc the cause of this condition, but, generally, it is a bend in the bridge that brings al]out X'ing of the rims. To determine whether this situation exists, the frame is held up from a side view with the sides extended. Using only one eye to avoid parallax, it is then determined whether both rims are parallel and in the same plane.

Fig.22.6 Plane of one rim at an angle to that of the other

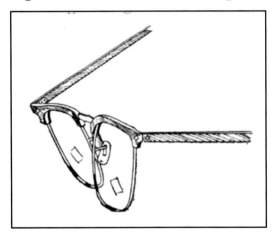

The fact that the sides are not parallel from a side view may or may not be an indication of rims **X'ing**. It is possible for the rims to be perfectly parallel and for the sides still to be not parallel. The easiest check points are the temporal border of one rim compared with the nasal border of the other, or the bottom of one rim compared with the bottom of the other. To remedy the **X'ing** of a metal or combination frame, the following procedure may be employed:

The inside of the frame is grasped at the juncture of bridge and rim with the thumbs, while the remaining fingers brace the nasal margins of the rims. The hands holding the rims are rotated until they become parallel from a side view [Fig.22.7].

Fig.22.7 Rotating the rims into alignment

An alternate procedure some-times used on metal combinations is to grasp opposite ends of the bridge with two snipe nose pliers or some similar type plier. It is better here first to wrap sticky tape or cloth around the jaws of the pliers, so that the metal

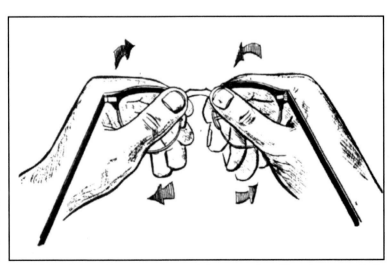

will not be marred [Fig.22.8]. The pliers are rotated in opposite directions until the rims are parallel.

Fig.22.8 Rotating the pliers in opposite directions until the rims become parallel

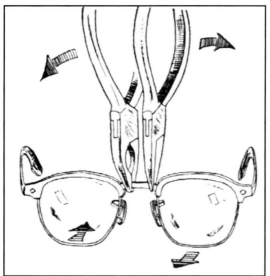

To rectify **X'ing** of a plastics bridge frame, the bridge area must first be heated properly until it is soft enough to be bent. Again the inside of the frame is grasped with the thumbs at the juncture of bridge and rims, while the remaining fingers are braced about the rims while they are rotated into proper alignment during the time that the bridge area is still soft. The rims still being held in the proper parallel position, the frame should then be either allowed to cool or immersed in cold water so as to "fix" the frame in that position.

Another problem of bridge alignment is presented when both rims are bent forward or backward from the plane of the bridge [Figs.22.9 and 22.10]. With a metal bridge combination, both thumbs are placed firmly against the nasal junctures of the plastics and metal rims, with the thumbs positioned diagonally. The first two fingers of each hand are wrapped around the nasal portions of the rims. Using an imaginary point midway between the thumbs [**x**] as a fulcrum, both hands are rotated about point **x** backward or forward depending on how the rims have been bent away from the

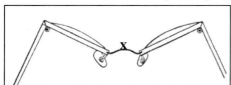

bridge plane originally. [This technique actually is used best when both rims have been bent forward from the plane of the bridge-see Fig.22.11]

Fig.22.9 Rims bent *forward* from plane of bridge

When both rims have been bent back from the plane of the bridge, as in Fig.22.10, the position of the frame should be reversed. Both thumbs are placed diagonally at the juncture of bridge and rims on the outside surface while the other fingers firmly brace the inside surface of the rims, and again the rims may be rotated into their proper plane.

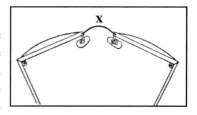

Fig.22.10 Rims bent *backward* from plane of bridge

Fig.22.11 Rotating the plane of the rims into the plane of the bridge

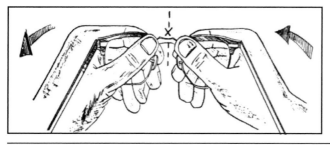

The plastics bridge combination frame is dealt with in the same manner, but first the bridge area must be heated sufficiently so that it becomes soft and pliable. Once the rims have been rotated into the proper position, the frame is immersed under cold water while being held in that position.

The lens planes should be not only parallel from side and top views, but also in the same corresponding plane with each other. Occasionally one lens plane is found to be anterior to the other while both planes are still parallel [Fig.22.12]. In a case such as this, two separate adjustments must be made to get both rims in the same plane as well as parallel to each other. First, a snipe nose plier may be used as a bracing plier to grasp one extremity of the metal bridge [A]. [This particular adjustment refers only to metal bridge combination frames.] Another plier of similar type, such as the hollow snipe, is placed adjacent to the bracing plier and is rotated until the opposite extremity of the bridge [B] is on line with [A] [Figs.22.12 & 22.13]. While a bracing plier holds a point close to the extremity [B], a second plier is placed at the very edge of the bridge and rotates the entire rim into the required plane. As in many other adjustments, it is possible to substitute the fingers for these pliers with equally successful results. Again care must be taken to brace the rims so that the pressure on the lens will not be excessive and result in flaking of the lens. In fact it is preferable to remove the lenses. The plastics bridge combination rimless types are handled in the same manner, but this time the fingers are used to brace the frame and move the rims into proper alignment.

Fig.22.12 Both lens planes parallel but with one lens plane anterior to the other

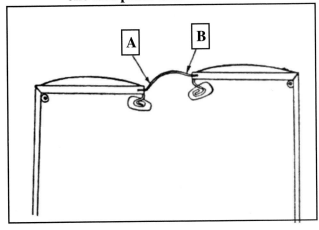

Frame Too High on the Face

By inspection, it is determined that the vertex distance is correct and that there is only the vertical problem to contend with. Multifocal wearers may report either discomfort or diplopia as a result of the segment being placed too high in front of the pupillary area. Whenever there is strictly a vertical problem - i.e., the frame sits too high or too low on the patient's face - the pad arms must be raised or lowered to bring about proper vertical positioning of the front. To bring the frame down to the proper height, both pad arms must first be raised, the amount being directly dependent on the distance the frame must be lowered. One suggested procedure is to grasp the top of the left rim tightly with the thumb, the forefinger firmly bracing the solder point area of the

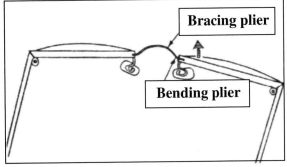

Fig.22.13 Bridge has been aligned-arrow shows direction in which rim is to be rotated

left pad arm while the remaining fingers firmly brace the lower part of the rim. For the right rim, the bottom of the rim is grasped with the thumb while again the forefinger is used to brace the solder point area firmly. The remaining fingers brace the top of the rim.

A parallel jaw or hollow snipe plier, held in the other hand, grasps top and bottom of the pad arm. Both pad arms are rotated toward the top of the frame [Fig.22.14].

Having raised the pad arm, the pad must now be re-angled in conformance with the standard pad adjustment requirements. The top of the pad, in this case, must be rotated backward while the bottom of the pad is rotated forward. To do this, a snipe nose or a hollow snipe nose plier is used to grasp the curl of the pad arm. The frame is still braced as shown in Fig.22.14. The plier then rotates the pad back to its proper position [Fig.22.15]. First both pad arms must be raised the same amount. Then the pads are re-angled. On certain well-constructed frames, pad re-angling may be produced by finger rotation.

Fig.22.14 Frame is properly braced while pad arm is raised

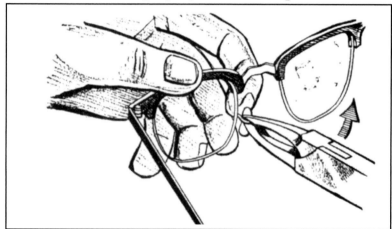

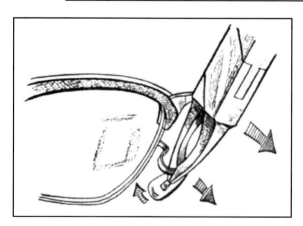

Fig.22.15 Rotating the pad arm back to its proper position

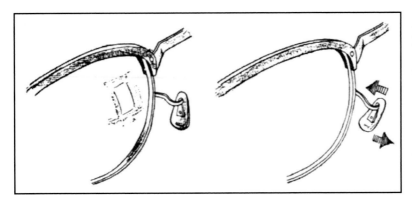

Fig.22.16 [*Left*] before adjustment

[*Right*] re-angling the pad

Frame Too Low on the Face

By inspection again, it is determined that, with the vertex distance being correct, only the vertical meridian of the lens plane must be dealt with. It may be noted that the top of the rim is below the brow, while the bottom of the rim rests too low on the cheek. Bifocal wearers may complain about having to raise the head in order to see through the segments, in addition to the myriad other complaints that can result with a problem such as this.

To raise the frame, both pad arms must first be lowered, taking care to brace the frame properly. [See Fig.22.14 for the proper bracing technique.] The pads must then be re-angled to conform to the standard pad adjustment. Figure 22.16 shows the change in the position of the pads that occurs when the pad arms are bent downward, and in what direction the compensatory re-angling must take place.

Frame too high and too far from the face

The bridge size of the frame-or, more accurately, the distance between the pads may be too narrow for the bridge of the patient's nose. As a result, the frame will rest too high and too far from the face. If the nose can be visualised as a three-dimensional triangle, the problem can be represented schematically [Fig.22.17]. It can be seen in Fig.22.17 that two points **AA´** resting on either side of the nose will, as a result of the wide distance between them, rest at a point close to the bottom of the nose as well as its base. Points **BB´**, however, with a much narrower distance between them, will come to rest at a much higher position as well as being close to the apex. This, then, demonstrates the mechanical principle involved when a frame rests too high and too far from the face because the bridge size [pad spread] is too narrow for the patient's face. This also shows why a frame rests too low and too close to the face when the bridge size is too wide for the bridge of the patient's nose. The terms *base* and *apex* in line. Fig.22.17 refer to the horizontal meridian.

To lower the frame and at the same time move it closer to the face, the pad arms must be removed apart, followed by a re-angling of the pads. The following technique may be employed to move the pad arms apart:

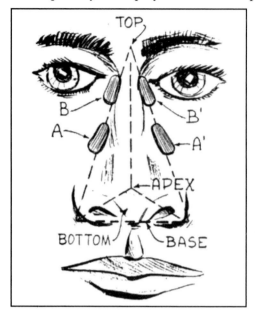

Fig.22.17 Potential pad position on the nose

While holding top and bottom of the rim and bracing the solder point area of the pad arm [as in Fig.22.14], a square-round jaw plier or a snipe nose plier held vertically is used to grasp the pad arm. While the rim is firmly braced, the plier rotates the pad arm outward [Fig.22.18]. Both pad arms are rotated outward the same amount. If a square-round jaw plier is used, the round jaw is used as the centre of rotation. For example, when the square-round jaw plier is used to rotate the pad arm outward, the round jaw is on the outside. When both pad arms have been rotated outward the same amount, the plier is then used to grasp the pad arm adjacent to the pad itself. This portion of the pad arm is then rotated inward so as to re-angle the pad [Fig.22.19]

This time the round jaw is on the inside, for it is again used as the centre of rotation. Figures 22.20 and 22.21 show a top view of a pad arms and pads as well as the position of the square-round jaw plier for each bend that is made. The directional arrows in Figs. 22.20 and 22.21 refer to the position to which the pad arm is being moved.

Fig.22.18 Rotating the pad arm outward

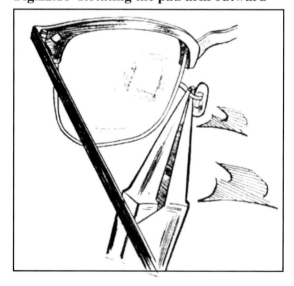

Frame Too Low and Too Close to the Face

To raise the frame and at the same time move it farther from the face, first the pad arms must be moved toward each other and then re-angled outward. To accomplish this, the square-round jaw plier may again be used, as was suggested in the previous problem. the frame is firmly braced once more, to prevent any flaking of the lens. The plier grasps both sides of the pad arm anterior to the curl of the arm, with the round jaw positioned on the inside. The square jaw is rotated inward about the stationary round jaw so that the pad arm is moved nasalwards. After both pad arms have been moved in the same amount, the square-round jaw plier grasps the pad arm adjacent to the pad.

Fig.22.19 Re-angling the pad

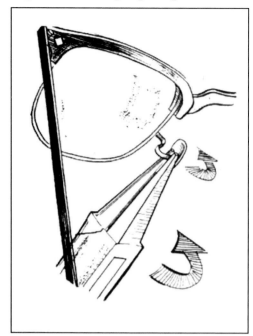

This the plier is so positioned that the round jaw is on the outside. The square jaw is rotated outward to re-angle the pad properly. Both pads are re-angled the same amount.

Frame too close to the face

It is often found that the front is positioned so close to the face that the lashes strike the lenses. To move the frame away from the face without changing the vertical position of the front, the effective length of the pad arm must be increased. The term "effective length" refers to the linear distance from the solder point to the pad itself, rather than the total length of the pad arm. The following procedure is suggested:

Fig.22.20 Before adjustment

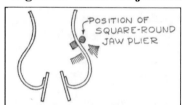

Fig.22.21 Arms bent out

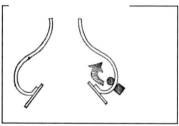

view:[*left*] **Before adjustment** [*right*] **pad arm straightened**

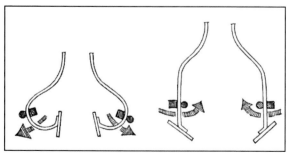

The rim and the solder point areas of the frame are firmly braced, as mentioned earlier. A square-round jaw plier held vertically, with the round jaw on the outside, grasps the pad arm at the crest [Fig.22.23, left] The plier rotates the pad arm outward until the pad arm becomes almost straight. The plier is then turned around so that the round jaw is on the inside, and at the same time it is moved closer to the pad than the original curl. The plier is rotated in until the pad has been positioned properly [Fig.22.23, right]. After one pad arm has been straightened, the other is then adjusted in the same manner. To maintain proper symmetry of the pad arm position, both pad arms **Fig.22.22 Top** *should* be given the same adjustment

before any new adjustments are undertaken. Figure 22.22 [left] shows a top view before adjustment; Fig.22.22 [right] a top view after pad arms have been straightened.

Figure 22.24 shows a top view of the position of the pad arms after the effective length has been increased.

Fig.22.23 Square-round plier in position to [*left*] rotate the pad arm outward and [*right*] rotate the pad arm inward

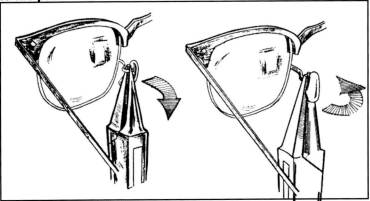

Frame too far from the face

Fig.22.24 Effective length of arm increased *top view*

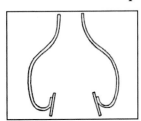

To move the frame closer to the face and yet not cause any change in the vertical position of the front, the effective length of the pad arm must be reduced. Here, however, it is not necessary to straighten the pad arm first. A square-round jaw plier may again be used, grasping both sides of the pad arm close to the start of the crest. The round jaw is on the inside and the square jaw is rotated inward so that the area of the pad arm concerned here is rotated both nasally and anteriorly. This reduces the effective length of the pad arm [Fig.22.25, left].

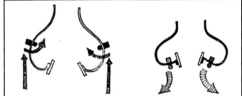

Fig.22.25 Square-round plier in

The square-round jaw plier may be placed at any point between crest and solder point, depending on just how close to the face the **position to [*left*] rotate the pad arm inward and [*right*] re-angle the pads**

front must be moved. Once the curls of both pad arms have been deepened, the plier then grasps the pad arm area adjacent to the pad. The plier then rotates the pad outward to re-angle it properly [Fig.22.25, right].

A snipe nose plier or a hollow snipe [parallel jaw] plier may be substituted for the square-round jaw plier in increasing or decreasing the effective length of the pad arm.

Front Too Far to Right or Left of the Face

This may be caused either by marked asymmetry of the bridge of the patient's nose, or by both pad arms having been bent to the right or the left. First, the position of the pad arms should be checked. If they seem to be placed centrally, it may then be assumed that asymmetry of the patient's bridge area is present. This is also then checked by careful inspection.

First, a case will be discussed in which the front rests too far to the right side of the face [Fig.22.26]. Let it be assumed here that the pad arms, through some mishap, have been bent to the left. This, of course, would be the cause of the front resting too far to the right side of the face. To move the front to the left, the pads must be moved to the right. The same techniques employed for moving the pad arms together or apart may be applied here. After both pad arms have been moved to the right, the pads are then re-angled if necessary [Fig.22.27].

Fig.22.26 Front resting too far to the right side of the face

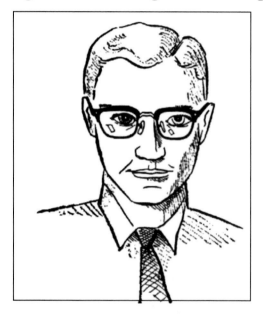

Assume, now, that the front rests too far to the left side of the face. This can also be caused either by asymmetry of the patient's bridge area or by the pad arms having been bent to the right. Either cause can be eliminated by inspection. In this instance, let it be assumed that the position of the pad arms is correct and that marked asymmetry of the bridge of the patient's nose causes the situation. Both pad arms would now have to be moved to the left, the distance being directly dependent on how much the front must be moved to the right to attain perfect horizontal alignment. Again the techniques mentioned for narrowing or widening the pad arms may be applied here. The pads must then be re-angled [Fig.22.28]. This illustrates the fact that, at times with a condition of facial asymmetry, frame asymmetry must be created to compensate for and thereby create an appearance of proper alignment. Many times facial asymmetry can be effectively camouflaged in this manner, provided that it is not too exaggerated.

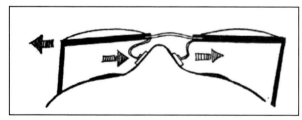

Fig.22.27 Arrows on pad arm denote directions in which they are to be moved

Fig.22.28 Position of square-round jaw plier: [*left*] before adjustment - pad arms centrally placed: [*right*] after adjustment -pads are then re-angled

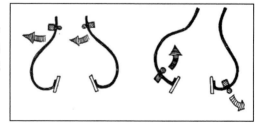

Pad Positioning

In any type of manipulation involving the pad arm, one must be careful to maintain the standard pad adjustment. This, however, is not quite enough. It must be noted carefully whether the pad rests absolutely flat on the side of the nose, as it should. If top or bottom or front or back of the pad cuts into the nose, then the pad position must be corrected. If not, the combined weight of frame and lenses can easily produce a sore area on the nose, the irritation being caused by the edge of the pad pressing into the skin. The pad should be adjusted in one meridian at a time until the pad rests absolutely flat on the side of the nose. Pad arm adjustments should also be taken in only one meridian at a time to insure symmetrical adjustments of both pad arms.

Adjustable Pad Bridges

The adjustment of pads on arms is most easily performed with pad-adjusting pliers, because such special pliers have a jaw that holds the pad securely without crushing the pad socket or attachment, and a jaw that holds the entire area of the face of the pad securely. The pad can be readily adjusted for splay, vertical and frontal angles by the use of these pliers. Snipe nosed or other flat-jawed pliers can be used, but unless used only on the supporting arm, they have a tendency to indent the pad surface. Once pads have been adjusted to fit the surface of the nose they should fulfil the following criteria.

- The pads should rest halfway between the crest of the nose and the inner canthus.
- The long diameter of the pads should be perpendicular to the floor when the head is erect.
- The full surface of the pads should rest uniformly on the nose. [Unless facial characteristics indicate otherwise].

Fig.22.29 Here the lower edges of the pads cut into the nose surface. This error can be detected by the U-shaped indentations visible after a period of wear.

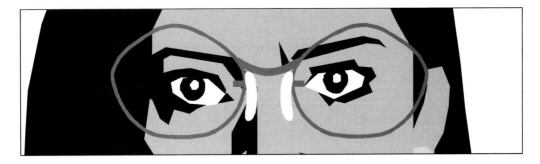

Fig.22.30 Here the upper edges of the pads indent the nose surface.

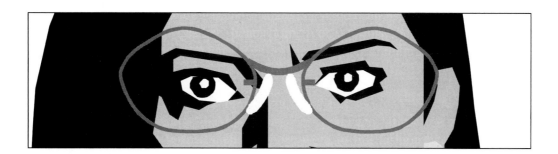

This can be checked by raising the spectacles off the nose and observing whether they fall back flat on the surface. If either the lower, upper, inner or outer edge of the pad strikes first or presses more heavily on the surface of the nose, the nose will show imprint or cutting marks after wear - or worse still may become too sensitive for continued wear. To correct these problems, the pad face should be re-adjusted as follows.

- If the lower edge cuts in - change the frontal angle by moving the lower edges of the pads apart [Fig.22.29].
- If the top edge cuts in - change the frontal angle by moving the lower part of the pads closer together [Fig.22.30].
- If the front edge cuts - decrease the splay angle of the pads [Fig.22.31].
- If the back edge cuts - increase the splay angle of the pads [Fig.22.32].
- If the cutting edge seems oblique, the pad is not vertical - alter the vertical angle and re-adjust to correct for one or more of the above errors.

Fig.22.31 This is an illustration of a pad splay angle which is too great [top view]

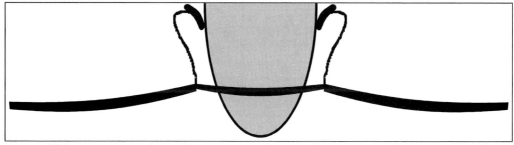

This may cause the pads to sit too close to the corner of the eye, especially in children.

Fig.22.32 Here the splay angle needs to be increased to prevent the back edges cutting into the nose [top view]

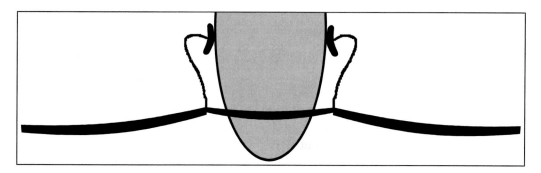

The Sides

When the front has been adjusted to your satisfaction and the criteria previously described for opening the side angle or let back angle, height, vertex distance and pad positions have been met, final adjustment is then made to the sides.

Heavyweight plastics sides are simply bent in the area behind the contact point with the head, above the ear. This is done in such a way that their broad surface lies fully against the portion of the head directly behind the top of the ear. The side must make contact with the head continuously from the top of the ear back, exerting uniform pressure all along that area.

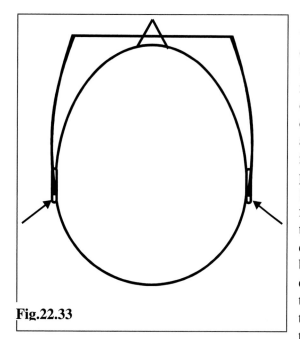

Fig.22.33

A common error is to bend the very last portion of the side so that the end exerts excessive pressure at a single point on the head. This type of maladjustment usually bows the rest of the side away from the head, displacing the upper part of the ear, and eventually digging a painful pit into the upper part of the mastoid process, where the tip presses [Fig.22.33 & 22.34]. When bent too far inward, the excessive pressure of the tips against the head causes the end pieces and the bridge to give, bending outwards. This in turn eventually releases the lateral pressure that holds the frame in position. For the inexperienced fitter, unaware of the source of error, the erroneous remedy is usually more of the same, which means increasing the side arc to restore the tip's contact. On the whole a vicious circle that finally results in widely bowed sides and excessively bent fronts [Fig.22.35].

If the structure of the skull is such that there is some convolution in skull formation, as is often found, heat the side and bend it to follow the convolution as closely as possible. The objective is to establish as much friction, through contact of the surface, as possible so that a 'disc-brake' action is introduced. If the frame front has been properly adjusted, the lateral side pressure correctly applied, and friction contact of the side well established, then the spectacles will not only remain in a secure position, but also will actually 'fall into place' automatically when put on.

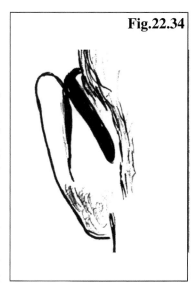

Fig.22.34

The proper lengthways position of the bend in the side lies just past the top of the ear, and the drop-end of the side should parallel the slope of the cartilage, comprising the auricle, but barely touching the cartilage itself [Fig.22.36].

Fig.22.35

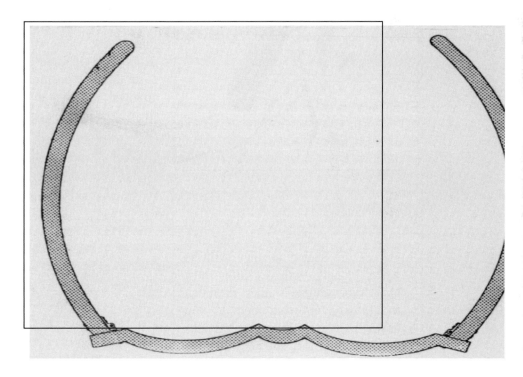

Above all, the side must not press into the crease between ear and head or the small chord of cartilage that helps in connecting the ear to the head [Fig.22.44]. Shape the drop-end to match the convolutions of the mastoid process, which is a lump on the side of the head behind the ear. It should exert even pressure throughout its length.

Side Length

If the sides are too long or too short, the position of the bend can be modified. There are of course limits as to how far the bend can be moved, since too radical a change will result in the drop-end being too long or too short. Plastics sides can be altered by applying the correct amount of heat to the appropriate point and re-bending. Metal sides can be adjusted in a similar fashion for minor alterations. If however the side needs to be shortened by a large or significant amount, then it will be necessary to remove the acetate tip, cut off an appropriate amount of metal with cutting pliers and then, after cleaning and smoothing any rough edges produced by the cutting, replace the acetate tip. It is also necessary sometimes to shorten the front end of the tip as well.

A metal side can be 'stretched' by a limited amount by again firstly removing the acetate tip and then relocating the bend. Thus leaving the reinforcing of the tip shorter than it was originally. Care must be taken not to bend the sides at this point.

Fig.22.36

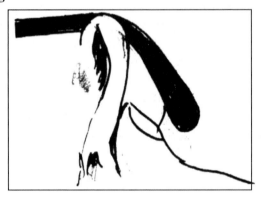

Since some side lengths are manufactured in increments of five millimetres, the prospect always exists that a side may not fit as precisely as desired on a patient's head. If this is the case, then the position of the bend can be changed, as it can also be in cases where there has been an error in ordering, or more likely, the unavailability of the correct side length. The suggested procedure is then as follows:

- Note the bend position - The front should be positioned so that the glasses are seated as they will be when properly worn. Often new glasses or sample frames fit much too loosely, allowing them to slip down the nose. When this happens the side slips forward until stopped by the ear. As a result, the bend appears to be properly situated, when in reality the sides are too long. To avoid this, with the wearer seated and the fitter standing, the fitter grasps the glasses around both dowel points [or lugs] with the left hand. He then gently holds them on the face in the desired position.

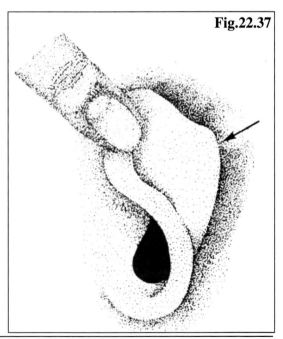

Fig.22.37

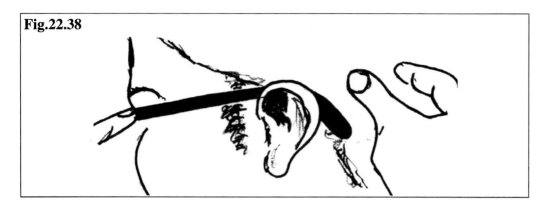
Fig.22.38

The right hand is then free to move the hair back or bend the ear forward to inspect for proper fit [Fig.22.38]. Although a discussion on personal space could provide enough for a chapter on its own I do feel that a brief word of warning is appropriate at this juncture. Whenever you touch a patient or their glasses or just move closer in order to take measurements or make adjustments it is strongly recommended that you advise the wearer of your intentions. Most people are then quite content for you to continue without being startled or shocked that their personal space is being invaded. Now to continue - for the left side, switch hands and repeat the procedure outlined above. It cannot be assumed that both sides will fit the ears correctly just because one does. Faces are not symmetrical. If the length of side is too long, the bend will occur beyond the desired position, which is just barely past the top of the ear [Fig.22.39]. This permits the spectacles to move forward until the earpiece rests against the cartilage at the back of the ear. It is possible to simply increase the bend in the side until the drop-end just touches the back of the ear instead of moving the bend. The fallacy here is that only two points of contact now exist - the top of the ear and the back of the ear

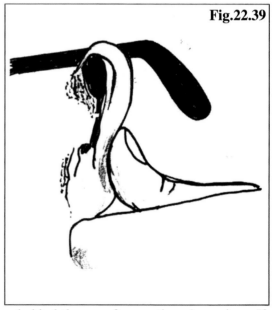
Fig.22.39

- resulting in an extremely painful place behind the ear after continued wearing. If the length of the side is too short, the bend will occur forward of the ear point, causing the drop-end to rest on the posterior slope of the cartilage. This usually has the effect of raising the sides up off the ear so that the bend itself is visible along the side of the head and the end of the side pushes against the back of the ear [Fig.22.40].

- Estimate new bend position - Observe the relationship of the bend to the position it should occupy above the ear and estimate a new position for the bend. Observe each ear separately as before.

• Heat both the original bend area and that portion of the side that you have designated to be the new bend. Hold the long section of the side firmly in one hand and grasp the shorter drop-end with the fingers of the other hand and gently but firmly straighten the side, avoiding the dreaded "double bend adjustment" Re-bend the side in the desired position by shaping it **around** the thumb or finger. Do not shape along the line of the thumb, as a sharp nail can easily damage the softened material on the inside of the bend. The drop-end should slope with its widest flattest part flat against the side of the head. It should be so shaped and convoluted as to follow the depression behind the ear [the ischium hollow] and the elevation following below it known as the mastoid process. There should be even pressure throughout the entire area [Fig.22.41]. The different properties of different plastics materials and the ways in which they react to localised heat and pressure are discussed to a limited degree in chapter 20, but the best way to gain this knowledge is by practical experience.

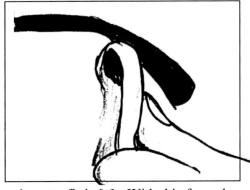

Fig.22.40

Curl Sides

These are used in situations where a hockey-end side will not hold the spectacles adequately, as for small children or for sports wear. The shape of the ischium hollow may follow several different contours [Fig.22.42]. The easiest shape to fit is [a]. With this form the curl side should not press against the root of the ear at any point prior to 'X' at the back of the ear. The curl should lie close to the root of the ear from this point to the end of the curl, since it is this contact that holds the spectacles in place. The very last 3*mm.* of the side may be turned away from the ear to keep the end from digging in. When the ear takes the form shown in [b], the curl should pass the point 'Y' without pressure before curling to grasp the balance of the ear. When the ear is shaped as in [c] the side should exert pressure on the ear only during the last 10*mm.* or 15*mm.* of the side length. This type is difficult to adjust, since the bend is almost at right-angles.

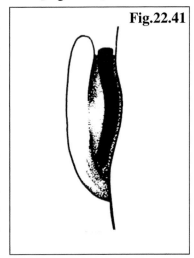

Fig.22.41

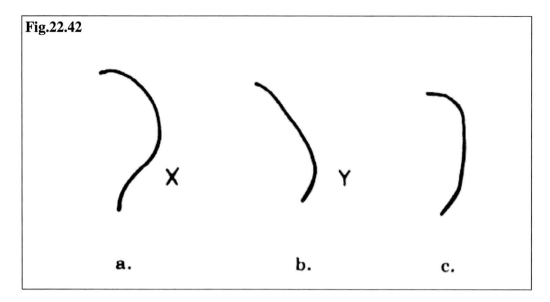

Fig.22.42

a.   b.   c.

Slightly long drop-end sides can be successfully adjusted to 'imitate' the firm fitting of a curl for children, without the usual loss of adjustment which often happens after a while to a curl side.

One Rim Higher on the Face

An example of this condition is shown in Fig.22.43, where the right rim sets higher on the face than the left. The possible causes are as follows:

    [1] the right hinge may be bent downward;

    [2] the left hinge may be bent upward;

    [3] the right side may be bent downward or the left side may be bent upward;

    [4] the right joint may be bent downward or the left joint may be bent upward.

Skull asymmetry could also cause this situation, with the right ear being higher than the left. With perfect skull symmetry of the patient, anything that will result in the right side being angled lower than the left [both sides being extended], will be the cause of the right rim setting higher on the face than the left. The cause is determined first by careful inspection of the frame and also by noting whether there is any apparent skull asymmetry of the patient.

If the hinge is at fault, it must be rotated into alignment while firmly bracing the frame until both sides line up from the side. For example, if the left hinge is bent upward, the left hinge and side must be rotated downward until the left side lines up with the right. The type of joint determines the type of bracing plier that is employed.

With a conventional type joint, a plastics joint plier or a fiberjaw plier, held vertically with the jaws pointing upward, grasps front and back of the joint. A joint angling plier, held horizontally, grasps top and bottom of the joint screw

Fig.22.43 Right rim higher on the face than the other

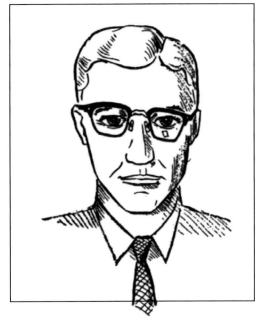

With the fiberjaw plier firmly bracing the joint area, the joint angling plier is rotated to bend the left joint downward so that the left side moves down to line up with the right. [For purposes of illustration here, the left hinge was assumed to be out of line-Fig.22.44.] To brace the joint of a frame having a trim attached, a soft rubber-jaw plier can be used. If the frame has a stone trim and it is impossible to grip the joint without having the jaws of the plier rest on the stones, the sides can be removed and the barrels of the front can be angled up or down as required.

Fig.22.44 Angling the left side

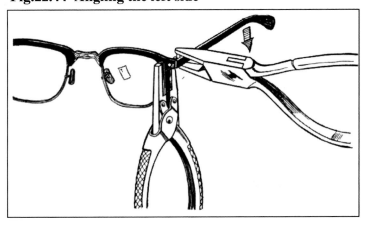

If the joint is of the curved type, a curved joint plier is used to grasp the joint and brace it. The joint angling plier is then used to grasp top and bottom of the joint screw and rotate side and joint in the necessary direction [Fig.22.45].

If the side proper is bent [in this case the right side would be bent down or the left side bent upward], the side would first have to be heated sufficiently When the side becomes pliable, it may be bent back into alignment with the fingers.

If a joint is bent and the lens is still intact, it should first be removed from the rim. The joint should then be heated properly; when sufficiently pliable, a fibre-jaw plier may be used to rotate the joint back into alignment. If both sides line up from the side and it is determined that skull asymmetry is causing the right rim to rest higher on the face than the left, either the right side must be angled upward or the left side downward until the frame sets in a properly aligned position when placed on the patient's face.

Fig.22.45 Angling the left side downward

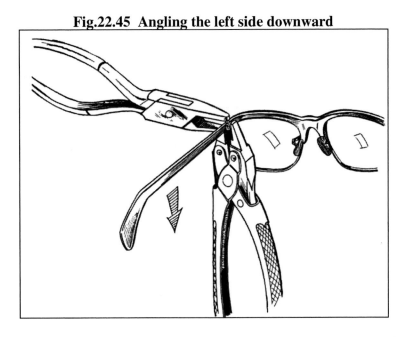

Again it is shown that, with facial or skull asymmetry, the part of the frame concerned must often be made asymmetrical to compensate and thereby create an appearance of alignment when the frame is placed on the face. If the left rim rests higher on the face than the right, the left side must be raised or the right side lowered, depending on the cause.

Fig.22.46 Improper side folding

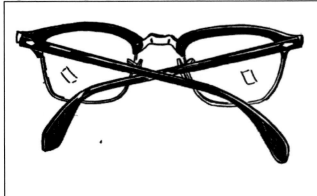

When folded, the sides should extend [in the plane of the rims] in a horizontal direction so that they are perfectly parallel. If, by chance, the sides are bent either upward or downward, they can be aligned by rotating the joint [in the lens plane] in the required direction [Fig.22.46].

If working with a conventional type joint, the following procedures are recommended: Thumb and forefingers may be used to brace top and bottom of the rim, particularly on the temporal side. A joint angling plier is then placed over top and bottom of the joint screw, and the side may be rotated in the required direction [in the plane of the lenses] [Fig.22.47].

For greater security, a fibber-jaw plier can be used to grasp the joint so as to brace the frame. A joint angling plier can then be used to rotate the side either up or down, depending on the direction required.   If working with a curved type joint, a curved joint plier is used as a bracing plier while the joint angling plier grasps top and bottom of the joint screw and rotates the joint in the direction required [Fig.22.48].

Fig.22.47 Rotating the side in the plane of the lenses

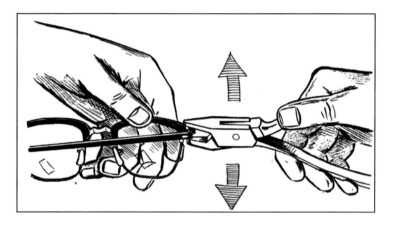

Fig.22.48 Rotating the side in the plane of the lenses

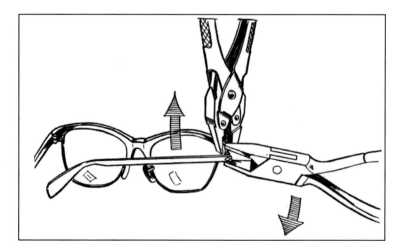

SUMMARY

In order to move:

Frame away from the face
- Narrow adjustable pads [also raises frame]
- Increase effective length of pad arms
- Shrink [narrow] bridge of plastics frame [also raises frame]
- Make front straighter

Frame closer to face
- Spread adjustable pads apart [also lowers frame]
- Decrease effective length of pad arms
- Stretch [widen] bridge of plastics frame [also lowers frame]
- Make front more curved

Frame off the cheeks
- Decrease the angle of tilt
- Raise frame by narrowing bridge or pads
- Increase vertex distance by narrowing bridge or pads

Frame higher on face
- Shrink or narrow bridge or pads

Frame lower on face
- Stretch or widen bridge or pads

One lens closer to the face
- If left lens is **IN** ————————————→ bring left side **IN**
  and/or   OR
  right lens is **OUT** ————————————→ bring right side **OUT**

- If right lens is **IN** ————————————→ bring right side **IN**
  and/or   OR
  left lens is **OUT** ————————————→ bring left side **OUT**

One lens higher on the face
- If left lens is **UP** ————————————→ bend left side **UP**
  and/or   OR
  right lens is **DOWN** ————————————→ bend right side **DOWN**

- If right lens is **UP** ————————————→ bend right side **UP**
  and/or   OR
  left lens is **DOWN** ————————————→ bend left side **DOWN**

23. ORDERING

When ordering a pair of spectacles it is important that certain guidelines are adopted in addition to those laid down by your organisation and the suppliers. There are also certain minimum requirements set out in BS 2738 Part 3:1991. If these are adopted by you as a regular discipline then misunderstandings leading to errors can be avoided.

One obvious and frequent source of errors is of course illegible handwriting. This has been alleviated considerably since the introduction of computerised ordering and dispensing systems into many practices.

On all prescription orders you must state the spherical power for each eye and also, where appropriate, the cylindrical power and its axis, the prismatic power and its direction, and the near addition if applicable. It is recommended that where one lens only is being supplied the above information regarding the other existing lens is also indicated thus enabling the prescription house to re-orientate the lens if there has been a need to remove it from the frame. It will also act as a safeguard in the event of a breakage.

Where the power of a lens exceeds five dioptres then the prescription should include the vertex distance at which the power was measured. This of course is not repeated on the prescription order to the laboratory, but the prescription is revised to take this and the actual fitting distance into consideration. Some computerised systems of course require both testing and fitting vertex distances to be entered and the necessary adjustments are made by the software program.

Most computerised dispensing programs will not permit you to continue with an order until sufficient additional information such as tint, lens form, material or type, have been entered. Obviously you must check that all of this has been done with a manual system.

It is usual to identify the data relating to the right and left eyes by the use of the initial letters 'R' and 'L', with 'BE' indicating both eyes for applicable data. The details for the right lens should precede those for the left lens. If the power is less than 1.00 then a zero must precede the decimal point and there must always be two digits after the decimal point. The degree sign [°] relating to the cylinder axis shall be omitted.

Where a prism element is included the direction can be indicated by the use of the words 'base UP', base DOWN, base IN or base OUT as appropriate. If the direction is an oblique one this is indicated by using the same axis notation as used for a cylinder axis, again omitting the degree sign. The directions UP, DOWN, IN and OUT can also be indicated by 90, 270, 0 or 180 [depending upon whether R or L] respectively.

Prescription orders will require the following additional information as appropriate - centration distance [monocular where eyes are asymmetrical], the position of the centration point *in relation to the horizontal centre line*, for multifocal lenses, the position of the segment or fitting cross *in relation to the horizontal centre line*, frame details or useable lens size. Some kind of identification code or provision for the details of the patient's name [address] as well as those of the optician. Plus of course the date of order.

It is recommended that, where single vision glasses are being ordered, the near addition is added to the distance prescription for reading glasses. i.e. not left as a distance R_x with an add. With computerised systems it is acceptable to enter 0.00 for plano sphere or the absence of a cylinder component. The following is an example of the lens details on a prescription.

R	Sphere	Cylinder	Axis	Prism	Base		Sphere	Cylinder	Axis	Prism	Base	L
I	+5.50	-2.00	10	2	down	Distance	+6.00			2	up	E
G H T	+2.50 Add					Near	+2.50 Add					F T

Vertex distance :   12 *mm*

ONE FINAL WORD OF WARNING, WHEN VERIFYING OR CHECKING COMPLETED SPECTACLES, ALWAYS CHECK AGAINST ORIGINAL PRESCRIPTION NOT AGAINST THE ORDER.

24. DEALING WITH PROBLEMS

A ll dispensing opticians will be faced with problems in their practice at some time. Indeed, most of us can expect to come across problems on a reasonably regular basis, no matter how good or how careful we are.

Problems may be easy to solve, such as a customer with an uncomfortable pair of spectacles, or they may be insoluble. Hopefully this last type will be a rare occurrence.

The problems we face may be with our customers or with our suppliers or with the prescribers whose prescriptions we are dispensing. We will look at each of the groups and their special considerations after we look at general problem-solving principles that we may apply to any difficulty.

Most of us consider problems, particularly customers' problems, to be a nuisance. Indeed, many try to ignore them or fob them off. The 'ostrich' approach, however, will only create more problems. Rather than look at them negatively, we should consider them as an opportunity.

If we can solve a customer's problems quickly and efficiently, it is likely to boost their trust and confidence in our abilities and our service. Problems, especially those of a technical nature, also give us an opportunity to use and extend our technical and professional skills. They can make life interesting.

Let's now consider the basic steps we use for problem solving.

DEALING WITH CUSTOMERS

Problem-solving: the steps

There are six basic steps involved in solving problems. If applied carefully most problems can be solved satisfactorily. In addition to a logical sequence of steps, problem solving also requires a calm and unemotional approach. A person with a problem may very well be angry and will vent their anger on you, regardless of whether you personally were responsible for their problem (you are representing the organisation they consider to be at fault). Their anger may well be in anticipation of a fight; that is, they may be expecting you to defend the situation. If you show that you understand their concern, you will significantly defuse the situation.

Step 1: Calm the customer

By being friendly, polite and actively listening it is possible to significantly diffuse the situation. Show them that you understand their concern without admitting liability. Also, assure them that you intend to find a solution wherever possible.

Step 2: Ask questions

By asking questions you are taking control of the situation. In addition to finding out the true source of the problem, it also helps to assure the customer that you are serious about helping.

Step 3: Listen actively and sift solutions

Listen to what the customer is telling you. They may give clues as to the underlying problem. They may also indicate what they think should be done. It is at this stage that you will consider solutions in light of the information provided by the customer (and any other relevant source).

Step 4: Recommend a solution

Once you have determined what you consider to be the best course of action, explain to the customer what you plan and get the customer's agreement. If the customer does not agree with your preferred solution, you have not yet solved the problem.

Step 5: Carry out the solution

Carry out the planned solution as quickly as you can. If possible do it while the customer is still with you. This will show that you are keen to solve the problem and to make them happy.

Step 6: Follow-up

Following up to see that the problem is truly solved and the customer now happy is an important part of problem solving. It demonstrates to the customer a genuine interest in solving the problem and in their welfare. The follow-up may be done immediately after solving the problem by, for example, asking them to now read a page with their progressives. Or, it may mean ringing the customer a few days later to check that all is now well.

This is a very effective way of showing your customer that you are serious about solving the problem. A successful solution to their problem and a friendly follow-up call a few days later will certainly instil confidence in you and your service; this is an important step in practice building.

Interpretation and memory

The problem-solving process must be applied carefully to avoid misinterpreting the problem. That is, we might set about finding the solution to an entirely different problem which, in this instance, doesn't exist. It is also important not to assume that the customer's interpretation of the problem is correct.

A customer may, for example, tell you that the glasses are too loose and are always slipping off when in fact they may be too tight, pressing on the temple, and the 'lemon pip' pressure is pushing them off.

Also, a customer may assume that because the glasses hurt behind the ear the bend needs to be adjusted, whereas the real cause might be that the let-back is uneven. See Chapter 22, which deals with many common customer complaints.

Remember too that memory, both the customer's and yours, can be unreliable. You may, for example, have said, 'The spectacles should be ready next week. I'll call you when they're in.' But the customer may have remembered, 'The spectacles will be ready next week. Call in and pick them up.' This means that the message sent is not the same as the message received. Whichever may be correct, it is the customer's perception that is now important.

If the problem is a technical one (for example, poor reading field in a new progressive), use your technical knowledge to consider the cause of the problem and the possible solutions.

Remember, whatever the problem and whatever the attitude of your customer, try to remain calm and objective. If your customer is angry or upset, part of your solution to the problem must be to calm them down.

The six steps in problem solving can be applied to any problem, not merely a customer's problem. It might be a problem with a supplier or a prescriber. More about this shortly.

Real and perceived problems

To all customers a problem is a real problem and indeed all problems require a solution. Unlike a real problem, however, a perceived problem does not require the obvious answer. Perhaps the best example is the customer who returns with a new pair of spectacles claiming, 'These are not the frames I chose; they're too large.' They believe that they have been given a larger frame because the spectacles feel loose. In such a situation it is not sufficient to simply point to your record card and say that it is the right frame. You will not have put the customer at ease. Instead use the problem-solving steps.

1 Reassure them that you understand their concern. Try to put them at ease.

2 Ask questions such as, 'Is the colour right?', 'If it sat higher on your nose would it look OK?', 'Did the frame you tried on feel firmer?'

3 Listen to their answers to your questions. Check the adjustment and find out why it feels loose. Also check all the other aspects of the spectacles, such as the positioning of progressive heights and how well they see through the lenses.

4 Indicate that you feel that there is a problem with the fit of the frame and ask the customer if you can adjust it to fit comfortably. You can indicate to the customer that when the laboratory makes up the spectacles the frame is often put out of alignment and in this case it may not have been realigned properly.

5 Adjust the spectacles and reinforce the improvement in the fitting. Seek confirmation from the customer that this was the reason that they felt loose.

6 It would be wise to ring this customer a few days later to confirm that they are still comfortable and that the customer is happy with the result.

Real problems, unlike perceived ones, are more straightforward. It might be, for example, that the segs are too low for the customer to read comfortably, or there is limited vision through the corridor of the progressive.

In some instances adjusting the frame may solve these real problems; in others it might require a remake. In any case the six steps in problem solving should be applied. The decision to remake or adjust would be made at step 4. Do not be hasty, though, many spectacles have been remade unnecessarily.

Common customer problems

Most customer problems generally fall within five different types.

Frame-fitting problems

These are problems with the frame chosen—that is, the frame does not fit properly. This is essentially a dispensing optician error and, if it cannot be remedied by adjusting the frame, will require a new frame (and quite probably, lenses).

Frame-adjustment problems

Without a doubt these are the most common cause of complaints, and they are usually fixed easily—or, at least, they should be. Adjustments are often underrated by dispensing opticians and optometrists. If you are unable to make an uncomfortable pair of spectacles comfortable after repeated attempts, the customer is likely to lose confidence in your skills and look for someone who can. Many, if not most, people are more concerned with the comfort of their spectacles than the visual comfort, particularly those with lower-powered prescriptions.

Service problems

These are typically complaints about late delivery of spectacles. The example quoted above in the discussion of problem solving is just one example. These are best avoided by taking care not to make promises, but, as our example shows, this is no guarantee.

Communication problems

The above example could also be considered a communication problem. Most of our time as dispensing opticians is spent communicating so it is not surprising that this is a source of problems. We need to ask the right questions and listen, not just hear.

Lens-dispensing problems

Lens problems might include poorly chosen lenses or lens treatments, or poorly fitted lenses. The latter might be corrected by adjusting the frame, solving such problems as segs or progressives set too low, or narrow field of view. Poorly chosen lenses would require a remake in most cases.

Whatever the problem may be, don't rush to remake the spectacles. Use the problem-solving techniques discussed above to determine the real problem and the best solution.

DEALING WITH PROFESSIONAL COLLEAGUES

Dealing with the laboratory

Like your dealings with your customers, your relationship with the laboratory is also commercial, although this time you are the customer. This is true even if the laboratory is part of your organisation; under these circumstances you are an internal customer. It may be more constructive, though, to consider the dispensing optician/laboratory relationship as a team. The better dispensing opticians do their job, the better the laboratory can do theirs and vice versa. Most of the problems that occur with laboratories are due to poor communication—poor teamwork.

There are two main areas in which problems between dispensing opticians and laboratories occur:

- communication

- quality control.

Communication problems

Before we can expect the laboratory to do its job, we must ensure that it has all the information in a way that makes it easy for it to process. This requires consistency and checking on the part of the dispensing optician. Many 'laboratory problems' are the result of unclear or incomplete instructions from the dispensing optician. The figures on written instructions must be very clear (some numbers can be easily confused) as must the signs (+ and −).

Another common problem is missing information: no seg heights or a missing PD, for example. The dispensing optician, as part of the normal procedure, needs to establish a system of checking all orders before they are sent to the laboratory.

Quality control

Most of the arguments between laboratories and dispensing opticians are centred on quality control. All laboratories should work on the tolerances in British Standards.

(some may have their own tighter tolerances). The most common arguments occur when the dispensing optician refuses to accept a pair of spectacles which falls within the standard. This raises a philosophical question, which this book cannot resolve. That is, should the dispensing optician (now with his or her customer hat on) require a standard that is stricter than the accepted national and international standard?

Many laboratories would argue that by being within the tolerances in BS they have met their end of the bargain. Dispensing opticians, however, may disagree. If the dispensing optician has made clear to the laboratory what is expected (their own standard) and the laboratory has agreed, the dispensing optician would have a strong argument.

If, however, the dispensing optician simply chooses to reject a pair of spectacles that meets BS but not their own strict standard, the laboratory may, justifiably, feel hard done by. The dispensing optician, of course, does have the right to change laboratories if they feel that the laboratory doesn't share their high standards. Once again such problems are best handled, if not solved, by sound communication.

It is important to remember that errors will occur even in the most efficient laboratory. Most laboratories have a fairly heavy workload and the person final checking may miss the odd incorrectly made spectacles. Equally, a busy dispensing optician may omit a PD or seg height in their instructions to the laboratory. Rather than leaping to accusation, it is better to simply address the problem and solve it. If the problems are consistent, a discussion with the laboratory manager may solve the problem—angst certainly will not.

Remember, too, that quality control works both ways. When ordering a pair of spectacles from the laboratory you must check:

- Is the lens (or lens blank) readily available or must it be ordered in? If you do not have an availability chart, a quick phone call to the laboratory will answer the question and save some embarrassment later.

- Will the lens cut out? Again, most lens manufactures provide a template for their lenses, particularly multifocals and progressives; use these charts to avoid a call later from the laboratory saying that the lens will not cut out.

- Is all the information on the order and is it clear?

- Have the lenses been priced correctly? Many jobs have been sent to laboratories, priced as stock lenses, only to find that a non-stock lens is required, and vice versa.

Dealing with the prescriber

As with the laboratory, the prescriber may be external to your practice or they may be associated (you might be working for an optometrist, for example). Again, good communication is important. It is essential when dispensing a prescription that you contact the prescriber if you are in any doubt at all about the prescription.

Problems are likely to occur in the dispensing optician/prescriber relationship where the prescriber feels that their instructions have been ignored or changed by the dispensing optician. A simple phone call will normally avoid such problems.

Whether the prescriber is internal, external or works for the opposition, it is essential that the dispensing optician not make any comments that could be taken as critical. Nor should the dispensing optician attempt to second-guess the prescriber's diagnosis (this really should go without saying).

If you do disagree with something the prescriber has said or written (they may have noted a different PD on the prescription, for example, or you may not agree with the recommended lens type), make no comment but talk to the prescriber in private and discuss the problem— tactfully!

CONSUMER RIGHTS

The law has created certain inalienable rights for consumers. These need to be taken into consideration when dealing with customers and handling complaints. Many consumers know their rights; it is essential that you do too.

A consumer has:

- the right to safety (that is, goods should not pose a danger to the customer)

- the right to do business without being defrauded (the trader should not misrepresent the facts or attempt to mislead the consumer.

- the right to equality in dealing with the trader (that is, the right to a fair agreement: a contract should not disadvantage either party)

- the right to be able to make an informed choice (a customer should have the option to choose what they want)

- the right to access a system of redress if their rights are breached).

In addition to these rights, consumer law also spells out certain obligations on the part of the trader in terms of the goods and services they provide. These are implied promises made by the trader. They cannot be waived by store policy to not give refunds or to only offer exchanges. The implied promises are:

- The goods must match the description. So, for example, if you say that the lenses cut out 100% of ultraviolet radiation, then they must.

- The goods must be fit for the purpose intended (assuming the trader knew the purpose—and it should be in the case of an dispensing optician). So, if the customer says she wants the spectacles for squash and you use glass lenses, you have not met your obligation.

- The goods must be of merchantable quality. That is, they must be fit to be sold. In addition to the obvious examples of 'unfit' spectacles (chipped lenses, scratched lenses, cracked frames etc), a likely test of fitness in the case of spectacles would be compliance with BS.

If spectacles do not meet the standards outlined in BS, they are not fit to be sold.

- The goods must correspond with a sample. That is, the frame the customer finally gets should be the same as the one they tried on off the display (unless a change has been agreed to).

- Services must be carried out with due skill and care. This would include such things as frame repairs.

The rights are not all in favour of the consumer, the trader also has some rights. Notably, the trader is not obliged to take goods back just because a consumer changed their mind. So, it is quite acceptable for a store to have a no refund policy, but it can only be applied when the consumer has no justification for a refund (such as, 'I just changed my mind').

Many large retailers, such as department stores, will, however, still offer refunds in such cases in the interests of public relations, even though they are not legally obliged to do so.

Summary

Many of the problems we are faced with are avoidable. We can adopt practices that will reduce, although not eliminate, problems. A thorough and systematic process when dispensing will anticipate and avoid most customer-related problems, as will care with our communication. In the case of problems with laboratories and suppliers, a strict ordering protocol will generally keep problems to a minimum. Established procedures for all staff in the dispensary and well-kept records are the best safeguard against problems. In the event that problems do occur, a well-organised practice should also have in place the procedures for dealing with them.

It is important to remember that communication is the key to successful dispensing. If we don't satisfy our customers' needs, they are likely to go elsewhere in search of someone who can. It has been estimated that only one out of twenty unhappy customers complain: the rest leave. Moreover, each unhappy customer tells eight other people; one in five tells over twenty people.

Be thankful for complaints, they are your opportunity to impress. If you are able to solve your customer's problem, you will win their confidence.

Appendix 1

In any cylindrical surface, the curvature varies from zero in the axis meridian to a maximum in any meridian perpendicular to the axis. In any oblique meridian that occurs between these two extremes, the curvature will have some intermediate value. For the purpose of calculating lens thicknesses we could express this curvature as the 'notional' power of the cylinder in any given meridian. If we denote it by $C_\square$ and the power of the cylinder by C, then

$$C_\square = C \sin^2\square$$

Similarly, the notional power of a toroidal surface of base curve B in a meridian at $\square$ from the base curve meridian can be taken as

$$B + C \sin^2\square$$

Table 1 gives values of $C_\square$ for cylinder powers up to 6.00D and for values of $\square$ at every 5-degree interval. It shows, for example, that a 2.50D cylinder with its axis at 65° [or 115°] has a notional power of 2.05D in the horizontal meridian.

Table 1. Notional surface powers of cylinders in oblique meridians

Cylinder Power [D]	Angle between oblique meridian and cylinder axis																
	5°	10°	15°	20°	25°	30°	35°	40°	45°	50°	55°	60°	65°	70°	75°	80°	85°
0.25	0.00	0.01	0.02	0.03	0.04	0.06	0.08	0.10	0.12	0.15	0.17	0.19	0.21	0.22	0.23	0.24	0.25
0.50	0.00	0.02	0.03	0.06	0.09	0.12	0.16	0.21	0.25	0.29	0.35	0.37	0.41	0.44	0.47	0.48	0.50
0.75	0.01	0.02	0.05	0.09	0.13	0.19	0.25	0.31	0.37	0.44	0.50	0.56	0.62	0.66	0.70	0.73	0.74
1.00	0.01	0.03	0.07	0.12	0.18	0.25	0.33	0.41	0.50	0.59	0.67	0.75	0.82	0.88	0.93	0.97	0.99
1.25	0.01	0.04	0.08	0.15	0.22	0.31	0.41	0.52	0.62	0.73	0.84	0.94	1.03	1.10	1.17	1.21	1.24
1.50	0.01	0.05	0.10	0.18	0.27	0.37	0.49	0.62	0.75	0.88	1.01	1.12	1.23	1.32	1.40	1.45	1.49
1.75	0.02	0.05	0.12	0.20	0.31	0.44	0.58	0.72	0.87	1.03	1.17	1.31	1.44	1.55	1.63	1.70	1.73
2.00	0.02	0.06	0.13	0.23	0.36	0.50	0.66	0.83	1.00	1.17	1.34	1.50	1.64	1.77	1.87	1.94	1.98
2.25	0.02	0.07	0.15	0.26	0.40	0.56	0.74	0.93	1.12	1.32	1.51	1.69	1.85	1.99	2.10	2.18	2.23
2.50	0.02	0.08	0.17	0.29	0.45	0.62	0.82	1.03	1.25	1.47	1.68	1.87	2.05	2.21	2.33	2.42	2.48
2.75	0.02	0.08	0.18	0.32	0.49	0.69	0.90	1.14	1.37	1.61	1.85	2.06	2.26	2.43	2.57	2.67	2.73
3.00	0.02	0.09	0.20	0.35	0.54	0.75	0.99	1.24	1.50	1.76	2.01	2.25	2.46	2.65	2.80	2.91	2.98
3.25	0.02	0.10	0.22	0.38	0.58	0.81	1.07	1.34	1.63	1.91	2.18	2.44	2.67	2.87	3.03	3.15	3.23
3.50	0.03	0.11	0.23	0.41	0.63	0.87	1.15	1.45	1.75	2.05	2.35	2.62	2.87	3.09	3.27	3.39	3.47
3.75	0.03	0.11	0.25	0.44	0.67	0.94	1.23	1.55	1.87	2.20	2.52	2.81	3.08	3.31	3.50	3.64	3.72
4.00	0.03	0.12	0.27	0.47	0.71	1.00	1.32	1.65	2.00	2.35	2.68	3.00	3.29	3.53	3.73	3.88	3.97
4.25	0.03	0.13	0.28	0.50	0.76	1.06	1.40	1.76	2.12	2.49	2.85	3.19	3.49	3.75	3.97	4.12	4.22
4.50	0.03	0.14	0.30	0.53	0.80	1.12	1.48	1.86	2.25	2.64	3.02	3.37	3.70	3.97	4.20	4.36	4.47
4.75	0.03	0.14	0.32	0.56	0.85	1.19	1.56	1.96	2.37	2.79	3.19	3.56	3.90	4.19	4.43	4.61	4.72
5.00	0.04	0.15	0.33	0.58	0.89	1.25	1.65	2.07	2.50	2.93	3.35	3.75	4.11	4.42	4.67	4.85	4.96
5.25	0.04	0.16	0.35	0.61	0.94	1.31	1.73	2.17	2.62	3.08	3.52	3.94	4.31	4.64	4.90	5.09	5.21
5.50	0.04	0.17	0.37	0.64	0.98	1.37	1.81	2.27	2.75	3.23	3.69	4.12	4.52	4.86	5.13	5.33	5.46
5.75	0.04	0.17	0.39	0.67	1.03	1.44	1.89	2.38	2.87	3.37	3.86	4.31	4.72	5.08	5.36	5.58	5.71
6.00	0.05	0.18	0.40	0.70	1.07	1.50	1.97	2.48	3.00	3.52	4.03	4.50	4.93	5.30	5.60	5.82	5.95

Appendix 2

Sags of lens surfaces

The exact sag formula is given as $s = r - \sqrt{r^2 - y^2}$ in terms of the radius r and semi-diameter y. If not known, the radius of curvature can be calculated from $r = \dfrac{(n-1)}{F}$ where F is the surface power for the given refractive index n.

Table 2. Gives the sags of lenses over a wide range of diameters and surface powers, the refractive index being taken as 1.523.

For a different refractive index n', the table can be used by multiplying the actual surface power F by $(n - 1)/(n' - 1)$.

e.g. a +12.00D surface on CR39 ($n' =1.49$) would be reckoned as

$$+12.00 \times (0.523/0.49) = +12.81D$$

This is the surface power which would be taken when using the table.

The edge or centre thickness of a lens can be estimated from the table by looking up the sag for a particular surface power and diameter and the adding the appropriate centre or edge thickness of the lens depending upon whether it is positive or negative.

e.g. a +18.00D lens with a knife-edge will have a centre thickness of 14.25mm at a diameter of 50mm. A −12.00D lens with a centre thickness of 1.5mm will have an edge thickness of 11.97 + 1.5 = 13.47mm at a diameter of 60mm.

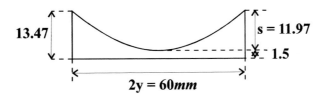

Table 2. Sags of lens surfaces at various diameters [n = 1.523]

Surface power [D]																

Surface power [D]	Lens diameter mm															
	46	48	50	52	54	56	58	60	62	64	66	68	70	72	74	76
0.50	0.25	0.28	0.30	0.32	0.35	0.37	0.40	0.43	0.46	0.49	0.52	0.55	0.59	0.62	0.65	0.69
1.00	0.51	0.55	0.60	0.65	0.70	0.75	0.80	0.86	0.92	0.98	1.04	1.11	1.17	1.24	1.31	1.38
1.50	0.76	0.83	0.90	0.97	1.05	1.13	1.21	1.29	1.38	1.47	1.57	1.66	1.76	1.86	1.97	2.08
2.00	1.01	1.10	1.20	1.30	1.40	1.50	1.61	1.73	1.84	1.97	2.09	2.22	2.35	2.49	2.63	2.78
2.50	1.27	1.38	1.50	1.62	1.75	1.88	2.02	2.16	2.31	2.46	2.62	2.78	2.95	3.12	3.30	3.48
3.00	1.52	1.66	1.80	1.95	2.10	2.26	2.43	2.60	2.78	2.96	3.15	3.35	3.55	3.76	3.97	4.19
3.50	1.78	1.94	2.11	2.28	2.46	2.65	2.84	3.04	3.25	3.47	3.69	3.92	4.16	4.40	4.65	4.91
4.00	2.04	2.22	2.41	2.61	2.82	3.03	3.26	3.49	3.73	3.98	4.23	4.50	4.77	5.05	5.34	5.64
4.50	2.30	2.51	2.72	2.95	3.18	3.42	3.68	3.94	4.21	4.49	4.78	5.08	5.40	5.72	6.05	6.39
5.00	2.56	2.79	3.03	3.28	3.54	3.82	4.10	4.39	4.70	5.02	5.34	5.68	6.03	6.39	6.76	7.15
5.50	2.82	3.08	3.35	3.62	3.91	4.22	4.53	4.86	5.19	5.55	5.91	6.29	6.68	7.08	7.49	7.92
6.00	3.09	3.37	3.66	3.97	4.29	4.62	4.97	5.33	5.70	6.09	6.49	6.90	7.34	7.78	8.24	8.72
6.50	3.36	3.66	3.98	4.32	4.67	5.03	5.41	5.80	6.21	6.64	7.08	7.54	8.01	8.50	9.01	9.54
7.00	3.63	3.96	4.31	4.67	5.05	5.45	5.86	6.29	6.73	7.20	7.68	8.18	8.71	9.25	9.80	10.39
7.50	3.90	4.26	4.64	5.03	5.44	5.87	6.32	6.78	7.27	7.78	8.30	8.85	9.42	10.01	10.63	11.26
8.00	4.18	4.56	4.97	5.39	5.84	6.30	6.78	7.29	7.82	8.37	8.94	9.54	10.16	10.80	11.48	12.18
8.50	4.46	4.87	5.31	5.76	6.24	6.74	7.26	7.81	8.38	8.98	9.60	10.25	10.92	11.63	12.37	13.14
9.00	4.75	5.19	5.65	6.14	6.65	7.19	7.75	8.34	8.96	9.60	10.28	10.98	11.72	12.49	13.30	14.15
9.50	5.03	5.51	6.00	6.53	7.08	7.65	8.26	8.89	9.56	10.26	10.99	11.75	12.56	13.40	14.29	15.22
10.00	5.33	5.83	6.36	6.92	7.51	8.13	8.78	9.46	10.18	10.93	11.73	12.56	13.44	14.36	15.34	16.37
10.50	5.63	6.16	6.73	7.32	7.95	8.62	9.31	10.05	10.82	11.64	12.50	13.41	14.37	15.39	16.46	17.61
11.00	5.93	6.50	7.10	7.74	8.41	9.12	9.87	10.66	11.50	12.38	13.32	14.31	15.37	16.49	17.69	18.97
11.50	6.24	6.85	7.49	8.17	8.88	9.64	10.45	11.30	12.20	13.16	14.18	15.27	16.44	17.69	19.03	20.49
12.00	6.56	7.20	7.88	8.60	9.37	10.18	11.05	11.97	12.95	13.99	15.11	16.32	17.61	19.02	20.55	22.24
12.50	6.89	7.57	8.29	9.06	9.88	10.75	11.68	12.68	13.74	14.88	16.12	17.46	18.91	20.52	22.31	24.33
13.00	7.22	7.94	8.71	9.53	10.41	11.34	12.35	13.43	14.59	15.85	17.22	18.72	20.39	22.27	24.43	27.02
13.50	7.57	8.33	9.15	10.02	10.96	11.97	13.05	14.23	15.51	16.90	18.45	20.17	22.13	24.43	27.26	
14.00	7.92	8.73	9.60	10.53	11.54	12.63	13.81	15.10	16.51	18.08	19.85	21.88	24.30	27.38		
14.50	8.28	9.14	10.07	11.07	12.15	13.33	14.62	16.04	17.63	19.43	21.51	24.03	27.35			
15.00	8.66	9.57	10.56	11.64	12.81	14.09	15.51	17.10	18.91	21.02	23.61	27.14				
15.50	9.05	10.02	11.08	12.24	13.51	14.91	16.49	18.30	20.42	23.04	26.71					
16.00	9.46	10.50	11.63	12.88	14.26	15.82	17.61	19.71	22.32	26.02						
16.50	9.89	10.99	12.21	13.57	15.09	16.84	18.90	21.46	25.09							
17.00	10.33	11.52	12.84	14.32	16.02	18.02	20.49	23.95								
17.50	10.80	12.08	13.51	15.15	17.07	19.44	22.66									
18.00	11.30	12.68	14.25	16.09	18.32	21.30	27.26									
18.50	11.83	13.33	15.07	17.17	19.89	24.37										
19.00	12.40	14.05	16.01	18.49	22.17											
19.50	13.02	14.85	17.11	20.24												
20.00	13.71	15.77	18.48	23.35												

Appendix 3

Compensation for change in vertex distance

Whenever lens powers exceed 5.00D attention should be paid to the vertex distance, that is the separation between the back vertex of the lens and the cornea. British Standards require this measurement to be stated on all such prescriptions and should be noted by the prescriber as the distance at which the trial lenses were used.

If the lens is subsequently dispensed at a distance different from this measurement the onus is on the dispenser to modify the prescription accordingly in order that the final lens will have the same effective power as the trial lens. There are several ways of doing this. In my opinion the most accurate method is by the use of a back vertex gauge and a table such as that overleaf or a similar one on a pair of concentric discs which allow you to align the power and vertex distance of the prescribed lens and then to read off on the scale the modified power at the new vertex distance.

Table 3 gives the modified power needed to compensate for a change in the vertex distance. If a plus lens is fitted closer to the eye or a minus lens further from the eye, its power must be increased. Conversely, a plus lens fitted further from the eye or a minus lens fitted nearer, must have its power decreased.

In the case of astigmatic corrections, each principal meridian must be considered in turn.

E.g. An aphakic eye is corrected for distance by +14.00DS/+1.50DC at 15mm from the cornea. If the spectacle lens is actually fitted at 12mm we need to consider +14.00D and +15.50D as the principal meridians moved 3mm closer to the eye. Table 3 shows that the modified meridians will be +14.61D and +16.26D. This means that the modified prescription to be worn at 12mm should be +14.50DS/+1.75DC.

Table 3. Modified powers to compensate for changes in vertex distances

Plus lens fitted further from eye or minus lens fitted closer to eye						Original power	Plus lens fitted closer to eye or minus lens fitted further from eye					
Change in vertex distance (mm)							Change in vertex distance (mm)					
6	5	4	3	2	1		1	2	3	4	5	6
4.85	4.88	4.90	4.93	4.95	4.98	**5.00**	5.03	5.05	5.08	5.10	5.13	5.15
5.32	5.35	5.38	5.41	5.44	5.47	**5.50**	5.53	5.56	5.59	5.62	5.66	5.69
5.79	5.83	5.86	5.89	5.93	5.96	**6.00**	6.04	6.07	6.11	6.15	6.19	6.22
6.26	6.30	6.34	6.38	6.42	6.46	**6.50**	6.54	6.59	6.63	6.67	6.72	6.76
6.72	6.76	6.81	6.86	6.90	6.95	**7.00**	7.05	7.10	7.15	7.20	7.25	7.31
7.18	7.23	7.28	7.33	7.39	7.44	**7.50**	7.56	7.61	7.67	7.73	7.79	7.85
7.63	7.69	7.75	7.81	7.87	7.94	**8.00**	8.06	8.13	8.20	8.26	8.33	8.40
8.09	8.15	8.22	8.29	8.36	8.43	**8.50**	8.57	8.65	8.72	8.80	8.88	8.96
8.54	8.61	8.69	8.76	8.84	8.92	**9.00**	9.08	9.16	9.25	9.34	9.42	9.51
8.99	9.07	9.15	9.24	9.32	9.41	**9.50**	9.59	9.68	9.78	9.88	9.97	10.07
9.43	9.52	9.62	9.71	9.80	9.90	**10.00**	10.10	10.20	10.31	10.42	10.53	10.64
9.88	9.98	10.08	10.18	10.28	10.39	**10.50**	10.61	10.73	10.84	10.96	11.08	11.21
10.32	10.43	10.54	10.65	10.76	10.88	**11.00**	11.12	11.25	11.38	11.51	11.64	11.78
10.76	10.87	10.99	11.12	11.24	11.37	**11.50**	11.63	11.77	11.91	12.05	12.20	12.35
11.19	11.32	11.45	11.58	11.72	11.86	**12.00**	12.15	12.30	12.45	12.61	12.77	12.93
11.63	11.76	11.90	12.05	12.20	12.35	**12.50**	12.66	12.82	12.99	13.16	13.33	13.51
12.06	12.21	12.36	12.51	12.67	12.83	**13.00**	13.17	13.35	13.53	13.71	13.90	14.10
12.49	12.65	12.81	12.97	13.15	13.32	**13.50**	13.68	13.87	14.07	14.27	14.48	14.69
12.92	13.08	13.26	13.44	13.62	13.81	**14.00**	14.20	14.40	14.61	14.83	15.05	15.28
13.34	13.52	13.71	13.90	14.09	14.29	**14.50**	14.71	14.93	15.16	15.39	15.63	15.88
13.76	13.95	14.15	14.35	14.56	14.78	**15.00**	15.23	15.46	15.71	15.96	16.22	16.48
14.18	14.39	14.60	14.81	15.03	15.26	**15.50**	15.74	16.00	16.26	16.52	16.80	17.09
14.60	14.81	15.04	15.27	15.50	15.75	**16.00**	16.26	16.53	16.81	17.09	17.39	17.70
15.01	15.24	15.48	15.72	15.97	16.23	**16.50**	16.78	17.06	17.36	17.67	17.98	18.31
15.43	15.67	15.92	16.18	16.44	16.72	**17.00**	17.29	17.60	17.91	18.24	18.58	18.93
15.84	16.09	16.36	16.63	16.91	17.20	**17.50**	17.81	18.13	18.47	18.82	19.18	19.55
16.25	16.51	16.79	17.08	17.37	17.68	**18.00**	18.33	18.67	19.03	19.40	19.78	20.18
16.65	16.93	17.23	17.53	17.84	18.16	**18.50**	18.85	19.21	19.59	19.98	20.39	20.81
17.06	17.35	17.66	17.98	18.30	18.65	**19.00**	19.37	19.75	20.15	20.56	20.99	21.44
17.46	17.77	18.09	18.42	18.77	19.13	**19.50**	19.89	20.29	20.71	21.15	21.61	22.08
17.86	18.18	18.52	18.87	19.23	19.61	**20.00**	20.41	20.83	21.28	21.74	22.22	22.73
18.25	18.59	18.95	19.31	19.69	20.09	**20.50**	20.93	21.38	21.84	22.33	22.84	23.38
18.65	19.00	19.37	19.76	20.15	20.57	**21.00**	21.45	21.92	22.41	22.93	23.46	24.03
19.04	19.41	19.80	20.20	20.61	21.05	**21.50**	21.97	22.47	22.98	23.52	24.09	24.68
19.43	19.82	20.22	20.64	21.07	21.53	**22.00**	22.49	23.01	23.55	24.12	24.72	25.35
19.82	20.22	20.64	21.08	21.53	22.00	**22.50**	23.02	23.56	24.13	24.73	25.35	26.01
20.21	20.63	21.06	21.52	21.99	22.48	**23.00**	23.54	24.11	24.70	25.33	25.99	26.68
20.60	21.03	21.48	21.95	22.45	22.96	**23.50**	24.07	24.66	25.28	25.94	26.63	27.36
20.98	21.43	21.90	22.39	22.90	23.44	**24.00**	24.59	25.21	25.86	26.55	27.27	28.04
21.36	21.83	22.31	22.82	23.36	23.91	**24.50**	25.12	25.76	26.44	27.16	27.92	28.72
21.74	22.22	22.73	23.26	23.81	24.39	**25.00**	25.64	26.32	27.03	27.78	28.57	29.41
22.12	22.62	23.14	23.69	24.26	24.87	**25.50**	26.17	26.87	27.61	28.40	29.23	30.11
22.49	23.01	23.55	24.12	24.71	25.34	**26.00**	26.69	27.43	28.20	29.02	29.89	30.81
22.86	23.40	23.96	24.55	25.17	25.82	**26.50**	27.22	27.98	28.79	29.64	30.55	31.51
23.24	23.79	24.37	24.98	25.62	26.29	**27.00**	27.75	28.54	29.38	30.27	31.21	32.22
23.61	24.18	24.77	25.40	26.07	26.76	**27.50**	28.28	29.10	29.97	30.90	31.88	32.93
23.97	24.56	25.18	25.83	26.52	27.24	**28.00**	28.81	29.66	30.57	31.53	32.56	33.65
24.34	24.95	25.58	26.26	26.96	27.71	**28.50**	29.34	30.22	31.16	32.17	33.24	34.38
24.70	25.33	25.99	26.68	27.41	28.18	**29.00**	29.87	30.79	31.76	32.81	33.92	35.11
25.06	25.71	26.39	27.10	27.86	28.65	**29.50**	30.40	31.35	32.36	33.45	34.60	35.84
25.42	26.09	26.79	27.52	28.30	29.13	**30.00**	30.93	31.91	32.97	34.09	35.29	36.59